Handle with Care

HANDLE

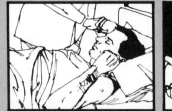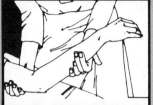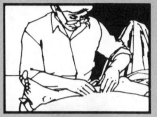

WITH CARE

A Handbook for

Care Teams Serving People with AIDS

Ronald H. Sunderland and Earl E. Shelp

ABINGDON PRESS
NASHVILLE

HANDLE WITH CARE

Copyright © 1990 by Abingdon Press

This book is printed on acid-free paper.

Library of Congress Cataloging-in-Publication Data

Sunderland, Ronald, 1929-
    Handle with care : a handbook for care teams serving people with
AIDS / Ronald H. Sunderland, Earl E. Shelp.
        p.   cm.
    Includes bibliographical references (p.   ).
    ISBN 0-687-16576-8 (paper / alkaline)
    1. AIDS (Disease)—Patients—Pastoral counseling of.   I. Shelp,
Earl E., 1947-   . II. Title.
BV4460.7.S87   1990
259'.4—dc20   90-750
                                                                                    CIP

Some illustrations in chapter 7 are adaptations from "Caring for Your Loved One at Home." Used by permission of the American Cancer Society, Texas Division, Inc.

MANUFACTURED IN THE UNITED STATES OF AMERICA

To the men, women, and children living with AIDS
who have invited us into their lives;
and
to the dedicated members of the
AIDS Care Teams in Houston, Texas,
whose loving ministries inspire us
and teach us the meaning and content of care.

ACKNOWLEDGMENTS

This book is the result of planning and guidance of the staff and consultants of the Foundation for Interfaith Research and Ministry and the Care Team leaders and members whose devotion to their task we gratefully acknowledge. We thank Frances Moncure for her counsel in the preparation of the basic nursing skills section of the text. We thank, also, Sue Cooper, for her contribution to the revision of material related to team structure, organization, and supervision. The American Cancer Society has graciously helped with the illustrations in chapter 7. Staff members Edwin DuBose, Pat Meister, and Tori Williams assisted in the final revision. Without their dedication, the ministry undertaken by the Care Teams would not have been possible.

We acknowledge with thanks and pride two groups of people. First, the patients for whom team members care, who have invited us into their homes and into their lives; they are our teachers. Second, we acknowledge the dedication of the Care Team members. Their ministry to people living with AIDS puts them on the front line, and they have not flinched from their service.

CONTENTS

PREFACE

In many ways, this book is a part of our personal stories. It reflects our individual and joint experiences, and the collective experiences of the hundreds of laypeople who have worked with us since 1985. Our work, and therefore this book, grows out of and builds upon our broadening and deepening appreciation for the complex issues that identify and prescribe ministry in "the AIDS era."

We are continually adding to our knowledge about AIDS ministries as we talk with Care Team leaders and members who participate in the Houston interfaith ministry program and meet with people in other communities around the country who have devoted themselves to the care of people living with AIDS. We are quick to acknowledge that our work is not complete, and this book represents merely a milestone on a lengthening journey. Or, to change the metaphor, it is like a still frame from a movie; the action is stopped momentarily so that what has been accomplished can be examined, but in another moment the film will begin again. More experiences will be added; new understandings await us.

What we present here, then, is not a definitive text but a descriptive account of how we provide AIDS ministries based on our experiences in the AIDS Interfaith Council in Houston. We are well aware that programs are emerging across the United States which bear a general resemblance to our activities, but which reflect the unique characteristics of particular settings in response to localized needs and opportunities. We offer this account in the hope that our experiences will be of assistance to other communities, will help interfaith groups develop AIDS programs where these do not yet exist, and will stir the hearts of members of congregations who are yet unconvinced that ministry to people living with AIDS is mandated for us as God's people.

This text does not include a model for AIDS education, although we assume that the provision of AIDS awareness materials and seminars is a vital prerequisite to the development of AIDS ministries. A starting point for many congregations will be the program resource departments of their respective denominations. Much of what is basic to AIDS education now exists in resources developed by religious agencies, judicatories, and secular sources such as the Red Cross and the Centers for Disease Control (CDC). Neither have we attempted to offer resources for the various ministries of clergy. We do not address premarital or other clergy counseling functions in the light of HIV infection, nor have we attempted to offer resources for the preaching ministry, although we believe clergy may find useful materials in this text and in our other books. Once again, statements and developed resources of the respective faith groups may prove ready sources for sermon preparation. These ministries will be addressed by us in a future volume now in preparation.

This book is a resource for congregations wishing to participate in an interfaith care program. We anticipate its use as a guide from which laypeople and clergy will gain insight for their work. The teaching sections are therefore in the format of an instructional manual, with appropriate major and minor headings. Nevertheless, our intention is also to provide information to a general readership among whom are people with a desire to care for people living with AIDS.

We believe from our own experiences and from discussions with other AIDS care-givers that each of us has a personal story to tell. Some time ago, a colleague in another city phoned to inform us that he had been invited to lecture on AIDS ministries to military personnel in Europe. Not having ministered to people with AIDS, he asked what he should read. We informed him at once that addressing AIDS ministry issues was not something about which one could read; the only basis from which to speak about AIDS was one's own personal experience in ministry. Perhaps, we suggested, one of us should go in his place!

Our colleague quickly stated he felt called to go to Europe, but needed help to identify a starting point. We suggested that he begin with people living with AIDS in his own community, who would teach him what he needed to know. Two months later, he phoned again. He had found people with AIDS and had ministered to them. More important, they had ministered to him. He had just one further question: once one has begun to minister to people living with AIDS, how does one extricate oneself from this experience. We responded that we had overlooked warning him that once the care-giver has taken up this ministry, it is often impossible to lay it down. One carries this ministry in one's heart; it becomes part of one's being.

Because this is such a personal ministry, it's appropriate for us to begin this text with a partial account of our separate journeys. It is our hope that the genesis of our personal pilgrimages and the means by which they merged will inform our readers and inspire them to set out on their own journeys. To people already toiling along this *via dolorosa*, a path along which joys are mingled with sorrows and pain, we celebrate your ministry, and with you offer all of our work back to our creating and redeeming God.

Terms

One of the issues in preparing this document was the choice of appropriate terminology in reference to the people we serve. With other care-givers serving people living with AIDS, we urge that such terms as *victim* and *sufferer* should be avoided. Terms such as *patient*, *client*, and even the acronym *PWA*, which depersonalize people, may be resented. Nevertheless, some term or terms must be used to refer to the people to whom this ministry is directed, in the process of reducing Care Team activities to some form of systematic presentation. *Client* will be used to refer to a person living with AIDS who is assigned to a Care Team, and *patient* will be used in reference to those activities associated with more physical care, for example, basic nursing care. *Human immunodeficiency virus (HIV) disease* will refer to the entire syndrome, including diagnosis as HIV-antibody positive, the psychosocial dimensions of infection, onset of symptoms, and frank or full-blown AIDS. *People with AIDS* will refer to persons who are HIV-antibody positive. *People living with AIDS* will include clients/patients, and the circle of people affected by the presence of infection in a family member or friend. For a medical classification of HIV disease, see Institute of Medicine, National Academy of Sciences, *Confronting AIDS: Update 1988* (Washington, D.C.: National Academy Press, 1988), pp. 202ff.

The terms *lover* and *partner* are both used to refer to gay relationships. They will be used interchangeably in this book, in deference to usages among gay men.

Our use of the phrase *families of people living with HIV disease*, or simply *families*, is inclusive. The tendency is to restrict family memberships to people related by blood or by legal recognition, for example, marriage or adoption. While we support fully these understandings of family, we also recognize other relationships of mutual commitment and care, such as those between gay men and unmarried men and women, that do not enjoy legal sanction, even though they respond to comparable needs and desires. Thus, when we speak of care for families, we refer to all the people who are related by choice or birth, are emotionally invested in each other, and mutually committed to care and support.

The term *care-giver* will refer to people engaged in various forms of pastoral ministry to people living with AIDS, whether full or part-time, or lay or professional. The term *care-provider* will refer to members of a client's family, lover, or other people who provide primary care to clients or patients.

CHAPTER ONE

Introduction

AIDS had emerged, by 1985, as a disease with unprecedented potential to destroy human lives, to disrupt relationships of every description, to reshape political and social agendas, to strain international relations, and to test the commitment of God's people to be agents of God's love. This dramatic, multifaceted threat is slowly being acknowledged by legislators, medical practitioners, researchers, and religious leaders. Since 1982, epidemiologists, scientists, and leaders in the medical community have sounded warnings accompanied by pleas for adequate resources to care for people with human immunodeficiency virus (HIV) disease and to find solutions to the catastrophic problems to which the human immunodeficiency viruses have given rise.

We became concerned, then involved, in the tragedy of AIDS in 1985; Shelp, through the diagnosis of Jay, his graduate assistant, and then with a growing number of people with AIDS; Sunderland, through daily ministry to patients in a clinic to which people with AIDS came for outpatient chemotherapy treatments and later as pastoral consultant to the Institute for Immunological Disorders, the country's first and short-lived "AIDS hospital."

Shelp's Formative Experiences

Through Jay, I learned my first lesson about ministry in the AIDS crisis: I learned that AIDS is *my* problem. I was drawn into a world that even now I do not fully understand. Neither do I know fully what to do now that I am in the midst of it. I am certain, however, that I must not flee from it, ignore the suffering, or refuse to try to meet the many challenges created by it. My certainty about these convictions becomes greater with each new person who invites me to be a part of his or her pilgrimage, a journey along which life and love can be abundant and enriching. My relationship with two other people during 1985 helped to clarify my ministry in an age of AIDS.

Gregg became my friend during his frequent visits to a clinic staffed by physicians specializing in AIDS. The clinic staff had invited me to be a consultant and observer. When Gregg came for his appointments we discussed a variety of subjects: his former work as a commercial artist, his carpentry projects at home, his commitment to his lover, his estrangement from his twin sister and other members of his family, and his Roman Catholic faith. It was obvious to us all that from visit to visit, Gregg was weakening and losing weight rapidly. More and more relatively minor problems were steadily stripping him of his will to live. He developed cytomegalovirus retinitis, which results in blindness, and was treated with a then experimental drug. Unfortunately, the drug made Gregg psychotic, and it was withdrawn. No other treatments were available. Clinic appointments were scheduled for him, but Gregg did not keep them.

I became concerned for my clinic friend. In particular, I worried about how blindness was affecting a man for whom an appreciation of color, texture, and shape had been so central to the value and meaning of life. I called his home repeatedly without getting an answer. Finally, I called his lover at work. Graham told me that Gregg had decided to die, that life was no longer worth living, that he was refusing food, had become incontinent, was too weak to stand or sit without support, and that he wanted it to be over. As we talked, Graham began to cry. I asked him if I could visit him that night. He agreed.

Upon arriving, Graham talked and cried for a long time. He knew of me because he learned from Gregg of our many conversations and of Gregg's sense that I truly cared for him. I asked Graham to ask Gregg if he would see me during my visit. Graham talked with Gregg, and then invited me into the bedroom where Gregg lay in the dark, clad in a T-shirt and diaper. Gregg told me of his desire to die and of his concern for Graham, who was exhausted and on the verge of a psychotic break. I didn't know how I could help except to offer to share in Gregg's care for the days between then and the time of his death. Gregg and Graham accepted my offer.

I knew that Gregg's care would require more care-givers than Graham and me. I called friends and asked them to help. Quickly seven of us became a team of volunteers doing whatever was required as, in turn, we stayed overnight with these two men who were alone and distressed because people who otherwise would have stood by them had withdrawn in fear. Day by day we watched in horror as Gregg's body wasted away. We watched his fleshless bones draw up into a fetal position. We sat in his darkened room talking with a man in a world literally darkened by his disease and marveled at his concern for his dignity, his sense of peace, and his desire for the grace of death.

Finally after our vigil of thirteen days, Gregg died. Only Graham was with him but the rest of us who became family soon arrived to share our grief, our tears, and to comfort Graham and one another. Through Gregg and Graham I learned my second lesson: that people can be moved to compassion and service when asked and when confronted with the horrifying, destructive impact of this disease upon people, the effects of which can only be compared to the obscenities of the Holocaust.

The third lesson I learned came from my brief relationship with Craig. For months I noticed this slim, handsome, quiet man who visited the clinic regularly. He was polite, never demanding, always patient, and seemed ever so gentle. There never seemed an opportunity to meet Craig until one day two weeks before he died. As we talked we developed an immediate and intense bond that I had not previously experienced. I took him home following his visit with his doctor in order to continue the conversation we had begun at the clinic.

Craig, I learned, was from the rural Midwest. He was part of a large family who knew he was ill, but were unaware of his diagnosis. One of his infections left him with neurological damage which caused him to experience periodic, uncontrollable tremors on the right side of his body. We talked for hours at his apartment. I returned the following day to find Craig too weak to get out of bed but wanting me very much to stay, to talk, to bathe him, to feed him, and to write letters to his family for him. He dictated brief notes to his father and mother and each of his grandparents. In each note, he told them he was having a bad day but that tomorrow he would be better; not to worry. Further, he told them with tears in his eyes and in broken voice that he had a new friend, a Baptist preacher, whom God had sent to him; with my care and that of Miles, his friend, he would be just fine.

A few days later when I arrived, Craig was in respiratory distress and his temperature was 105°. I summoned a friend and we rushed him to the hospital to be admitted for the last time. We called Miles, who came after work to Craig's side, and did not leave until Craig died. Efforts to save Craig's life proved unavailing, and both Craig and we knew it. I called his parents, who arrived thirty-six hours before Craig died. During the drive from the airport I talked with this humble, devoted, religious couple about Craig and discovered that they suspected but did not know that Craig was gay, that Miles was his lover, and that his illness was AIDS.

We arrived at the hospital at midnight and left Craig and his parents alone. It was difficult for Craig to talk. His breathing was labored and painful, but he was determined that they learn of his wishes for his meager estate before they left. After getting this business out of the way, Craig slept, and his parents went to a nearby hotel to rest. Miles and I stayed with Craig, one sleeping while the other attended to Craig.

When Craig's parents arrived early the next morning his condition had grown worse. But now Craig wanted to hear about home and family. No more talk about death. Between gasps for breath he tried to participate in this process of catching up with family. The pain-killing drugs and his weakened body interrupted this process with periods of restless sleep. About an hour before he died, he awoke, and only I was with him. I wiped his brow, brushed his dark, wet hair with my hand, and tried to assure him that his pain would soon be over. With great difficulty, he turned his head from side to aside and in despair said four words: "Earl, I can't breathe." His beautiful, hazel eyes reflected his love and trust, yet revealed terror that intensified the pain of this moment for both of us.

I felt inexpressibly desperate and impotent. I wanted to ease his breathing, to relieve his pain, and to make him better so that we could enjoy one another longer. But I could not. As we looked deeply into each other's soul with tears streaming down our cheeks, I began to understand better the rage that accompanies impotence in situations of injustice. I began to understand in a finite way how surely God felt as Jesus's life was unjustly and painfully being taken from him, and God could do nothing other than affirm the power of love by being there.

About an hour later, with Miles at his side, Craig's struggle was over. Craig's last message to me, in which more was communicated than a mere four words, taught me a third formative lesson for AIDS ministry. As individuals and as a community of faith we do not have the power to cure AIDS or any other disease. But the lesson my experience with Craig taught me is that we are not without resources and that we are not totally impotent. We are embodiments of love, empowered by God whom we characterize as love, and called to be agents of God's love for all humanity. The question before us as God's people is whether we will freely give the love that we have freely received. If we will do so in the midst of AIDS, we, the people of God, will relieve some of the suffering caused by AIDS and we will be an example for others to follow. More important, however, we will be privileged to have relationships, to enrich each other's lives, and experience joys and blessings without which our lives would be impoverished.

Sunderland's Journey

My visits to outpatient clinics in 1985 were assigned as part of a research project to identify and describe how pastoral visits in outpatient clinics differ from pastoral care to inpatients, in order to develop a ministry which had largely been overlooked by hospital departments of pastoral care. At first, patients receiving chemotherapy related to AIDS disorders were but one group among other groups of patients. As their numbers grew and I began to monitor their frequent clinic visits it became clear that, almost invariably, they were young, bright men whose professional and personal lives were gravely threatened by a new insidious disease.

In 1986, I participated in two life-changing events. The Institute for Immuniological Disorders was established as a facility dedicated solely to care for people living with AIDS and to research into HIV disease. I began a part-time ministry as pastoral consultant to the "AIDS hospital," and was drawn into much closer contact with patients, their families, and the hospital staff, including both patient care and research personnel. I began to experience the grief of patients as they learned from physicians that their illness was fatal; of parents who stood by, powerless to avert death; of physicians, nurses, social workers, and other staff whose best efforts were powerless to halt the ultimate ravages of this deadly virus. The hospital became a haven for people suffering from HIV infection, and a community of both grief and a remarkable sense of loving care which drew us together into one large family.

There were few instances in which ministry to patients did not include care for their families of origin, partners, and families of choice. Within this community drawn together by the onset of the AIDS epidemic, individual families often found themselves thrust with sudden, brutal force into a strange, alien world for which they were often totally unprepared. Alan's parents had been summoned to Houston from a small, rural village in central Louisiana. They were afraid, and at first we were powerless to comfort them. They had learned on arrival at the hospital that their son was gay and that he was desperately ill with a disease that would destroy him. Nothing in their previous experience had prepared them for the situation in which he and they found themselves. They were simple folk who had lived their quiet lives, were respected by their neighbors, attended Mass each Sunday, and were known by all as hard-working, deeply pious people whose values reflected those of rural America. I learned from Alan's father something of what life is like in such a community. He told me that the town boasted of one traffic light: "It isn't really necessary," he said, "because the traffic isn't that heavy. We don't have rush-hour, but it is handy to be able to say to visiting families: 'Turn right at the light, and our street is the third on the left'!" Alan's parents shared with me their terror at being forced to drive on Houston's freeways. The motel in which they were staying was run down, but it was the nearest motel they could find; they were afraid to drive a greater distance.

I learned that, in addition to their fears for Alan, they feared for themselves. "We have party lines in our town, so there is no privacy. News travels quickly. We had hoped that no one would learn which hospital Alan is in. But today we received two phone calls here. I guess everyone knows by now. Our's is the sort of town in which people feel they have a right to know what is going on in each family. If you don't get to the mail first, the neighbors are just as likely to open letters, then tell you the content when you arrive home!" The conversation was leading up to their own private horror: How could they return to their home after Alan's death? Would their neighbors shun them? And would they feel welcomed at Mass the following Sunday?

John's parents, like many others, were overwhelmed by his illness and his gay lifestyle. His mother refused to enter his hospital room while his lover, Stan, was present. The struggle continued for three days as John lay dying, yet attempting to accomplish reconciliation between his partner and his parents. We watched helplessly as the relationship between John's parents shattered on the rocks of their grief and despair. John's father tried to mediate between his wife and John, but to no avail. The day before John died, he said bitterly to his wife: "As I watch John and Stan, I am learning what love is really about!"

Max was a twenty-nine-year-old patient alienated from his parents, who had not visited him during his ten-year residence in Houston; there had been few family contacts and little communication. I sat with Max as he phoned his mother to tell her he was very ill and might not live. He pleaded with her to bring his father for a brief visit. She indicated she might be able to make the trip, but that his father would not come. As her arrival time grew daily closer Max became more anxious. Would she even come? What would they talk about? How long would she stay? Perhaps it would be better if he called her back and asked her not to visit him.

On the morning she was due to arrive, Max's anxiety climbed. He rehearsed with me what he might say. A social worker met her in the hospital lobby and for almost an hour she would not step into the elevator. Finally coaxed to Max's floor, she was unable to enter the room, immobilized by her fear of contamination from Max's infection. She moved to the end of Max's bed, then, with great reluctance, touched his hand only to immediately drawback. It was the only physical contact she had with Max before she left Houston the following day. Neither she nor Max's father made any further attempt to talk with him before his death, two weeks later.

Mike was more fortunate. His mother left her employment in another state and his sister interrupted her university study to set up home in Houston so that they could express their love for him. They remained with him through the early period, when the company for which he worked locked him out of the office building, through countless bouts of illness and hospitalizations, as he lost half his body weight, and were at his side when he died.

Pastoral relationships with families shattered by the tragedy of AIDS have led me to encounters with suffering at depths I had not previously experienced. There are moments of unspeakable sadness when words will not come, when words themselves seem an intrusion upon the private suffering and anguish of people, and silence is the only language capable of expressing the depth of shared grief.

The second life-changing event for me was Earl's suggestion that, in light of the failure of the religious community to respond to the growing AIDS crisis and the continuing ignorance of the nature and scope of the impact of AIDS on people infected by the AIDS virus, it was time to write the stories of people suffering because of this disease.[1] We are aware that the stories and our ministries presented in our earlier books were devoted initially to gay men who were living with AIDS. This reflected the Houston scene, where in the early to mid-eighties we saw few intravenous drug users, hemophiliacs, women, or children with HIV infections. That situation has now changed, and this book reflects our growing ministry to drug users, hemophiliacs, and families caring for children with AIDS. We have learned many of the lessons HIV disease teaches as we listened to patients and family members and recorded their stories, which stand as memorials to them and the growing crowd of witnesses to the uncertain world of AIDS. We have learned through our ministries since 1985, for example, what Thomas Ogletree means by his model of the church as a place of hospitality to strangers, where the people of God should be filled with a wish to protect the "stranger," that is, the vulnerable and the oppressed, in their struggle for liberation. As God's people, we must recognize the profound vulnerability of the oppressed and respond to their suffering with compassion.[2]

I remember vividly sitting with Ralph and Thelma, as tearfully they shared the story of their discovery that Ralph Jr., their only son, was "different," and that he had contracted AIDS, a double blow to this charismatic couple so embedded in the theology and practices of their pentecostal congregation. They told of their pilgrimage from closed, angry rejection of homosexuality, through bewilderment on learning that Ralph Jr. was gay (they could never bring themselves to use this term), to acceptance of Ralph Jr. and his lover and their friends whom they welcomed into their home and learned to love.

Interviews with other parents followed. Always there were the questions, doubts, and confusions, and nearly always the searching for theological assurances by parents who felt no reassurance except on one central issue. Each in his or her own way was strengthened by the conviction that love always triumphs over hate and ignorance, even death, and that God's love is fully able to accomplish victories to which mere mortals can only look forward with hope.[3]

Our Paths Merge

In September 1985, *The Christian Century* published our article, "AIDS and the Church."[4] We took the religious community to task for its failure to respond with urgency to the AIDS epidemic, only to turn and ask ourselves: "So what more should *we* be doing?" In January 1986, we sponsored an AIDS seminar at South Main Baptist Church, Houston, followed by the creation of an informal consortium of pastors and rabbis from which the ministry project ultimately evolved. By fall 1986, ministry to individual patients and families was being offered. The book of stories had been published and was being read widely.

We began to receive inquiries from Houston clergy asking how they could have a more active role. The model established by Shelp in ministry with Gregg and Graham, and Craig, his parents, and lover seemed an answer. The team concept was born (Shelp's first team called themselves familiarly the "Mary Magdalene Mission Squad"[5]). One by one, congregations were invited to establish what were then titled "respite teams," and more recently "Care Teams."

By the end of 1986, six congregation-based teams were in place, and 90 people with AIDS had received care in the few months the teams had been in existence. During 1987, five more teams were added, and by December 1988, the total reached 19, with over 300 laypeople involved. During a visit by then Surgeon General C. Everett Koop in May 1988, the name of the organization was changed to AIDS Interfaith Council to reflect the contribution of lay care givers. In September 1988, the Foundation for Interfaith Research and Ministry (FIRM) was incorporated to provide an institutional structure for the

Council's ministry. By December 1989, 30 teams totalling over 600 members were caring for 100 people living with AIDS.

Dr. Koop summarized the contribution of the Interfaith Care Team program when he stated: "What you have done here is absolutely tremendous. . . . You're way ahead of the rest of the country. . . . If it would be possible to take what you have done to other parts of the country, we would see such networks as you have here spring up all over the land."[6] This wish is now being realized, as forms of the Care Team concept are introduced in New Orleans, San Antonio, Little Rock, Corpus Christi, Albuquerque, Sacramento, Grand Rapids, Chapel Hill, Kansas City, Missouri, and other cities as a result of our visits to these centers and through the individual efforts of concerned people who have consulted with us.

Uses of This Book

Our thought in designing this text was not to prepare a book that would be followed to the letter, but to include a variety and depth of materials from which teachers might select. Service training programs typically are formed from training materials that are presented according to the particular interests and experiences of the instructor, the objectives of the program, and the needs and aptitudes of trainees. An outline of a typical seven hour orientation session for Care Teams assigned to adult clients is provided in appendix 1. An additional outline used with teams to whom pediatric AIDS clients are assigned is included in the same appendix.

Inquiries are invited from congregations and care-givers interested to learn more about the Care Team program. These should be addressed to Foundation for Interfaith Research and Ministry, P.O, Box 20528, Houston, TX 77225. Also available is a custom-designed, IBM-compatible software package to manage data regarding volunteer and team activities, as well as demographic and service data on clients. Requests for specifications and costs should also be directed to FIRM.

NOTES

1. Earl E. Shelp, Ronald H. Sunderland, and Peter Mansell, *AIDS: Personal Stories in Pastoral Perspective* (New York: The Pilgrim Press, 1986).
2. Thomas W. Ogletree, *Hospitality to Strangers* (Philadelphia: Fortress Press, 1985), pp. 2 ff.
3. See 1 Cor. 13.
4. Earl E. Shelp and Ronald H. Sunderland, "AIDS and the Church," *The Christian Century* (September 5-12, 1985), pp. 797-99.
5. Mary of Magdala is presented by Luke as a model of discipleship and practical ministry. Her identification as a harlot by tradition is not supported by scripture. See E. P. Blair, "Mary of Magdala," *The Interpreter's Dictionary of the Bible*, Vol. 3 (Nashville: Abingdon Press, 1962), pp. 288-90.
6. Ruth SoRelle, "Koop Praises Religious AIDS Support Here," *Houston Chronicle* (May 8, 1988), Section 1, p. 33.

CHAPTER TWO

An Interfaith Response to People Living with AIDS

Mission

The AIDS Interfaith Council[1] is dedicated to befriending and serving people living with HIV disease. The care offered by the Care Teams affiliated with the council is non-judgmental, and seeks to represent the ministry of compassion and acceptance that people of God are called to express. Members of Care Teams view themselves as friends to people they serve. Their service activities include:

Social, emotional, and spiritual support;
household tasks, including preparing and serving meals;
shopping and transportation;
assisting family members;
basic nursing care;
other needs as appropriate.

This handbook is designed to assist members of congregations who have committed themselves to a ministry of healing and reconciliation in response to the crises generated by progressive HIV disease. It suggests plans for the development of congregational Care Teams, including the training of Care Team members who, as representatives of the people of God, are called upon to undertake ministry to people living with AIDS.

The Care Team program is a two-dimensional ministry. First, it will be assumed that the most effective response in each community will be an interfaith effort that draws strength from the available resources in congregations and communities in the service of people living with AIDS. Second, while this service to people with AIDS is the first goal of the ministry program, such efforts are also educational in nature. The Care Team concept thus affords communities a unique opportunity to extend AIDS-awareness efforts so that accurate information concerning HIV disease can be widely disseminated, perhaps leading to a reduction of behaviors that place people at risk for HIV infection.

The project described here has been developed as a manifestation of the religious community's commitment to care for people with HIV-related diseases. Caring and compassionate ministry to people in crisis is one of the most fundamental characteristics of the people of God. The needs of people constitute a call to God's people to respond with love: We are to love our neighbors as ourselves. Ministry to people living with AIDS is but one channel for that love. In the current crisis created by progressive HIV disease, we dare not ignore the pain and anguish of people suffering from its impact.

In the years following the appearance of the epidemic in 1980-81, the blood banks, scientists and researchers, governments, health educators, media, and public health officials were tragically tardy in their response.[2] It should be noted that religious communities also were belated in their responses.

That tide is now turning, and congregations across the United States are in the forefront of AIDS programs providing hands-on, personal care for people living with AIDS, a term that encompasses everyone: people infected by HIV, their families, friends, lovers or partners, acquaintances, employers and colleagues, neighbors, health care providers, the communities of which they are members, and the congregations in which they find expression of their religious needs. The interfaith Care Team program is becoming the most widely used concept in the design of responses by the religious community to the AIDS crisis.

Care Teams may consist of as few as 8-10 members, but ideally 14 or more people. Members are recruited in congregations in which members commit themselves to a direct, "hands-on" response to the needs of people living with HIV disease and to coordinate this program with those of community social service agencies. This handbook is prepared to assist such interfaith programs.

Importance of Interfaith Ministries

There are many occasions and many reasons that lead groups of congregations to develop joint programs. Rarely has there been a time when such common efforts are so critical than that occasioned by the AIDS epidemic. The uniting of resources of individual congregations in an interfaith ministry of AIDS awareness education and care for people living with AIDS 1) represents the common commitment to ministry of participating faith groups; 2) maximizes the resources each group brings; and 3) offers a model for whole communities to follow.

1. Common Commitment to Ministry

The East Asia Christian Conference, an ecumenical gathering of national churches and religious bodies, called upon its members during the 1960s to commit themselves to "joint action for mission." It was proposed that, as a minority in a predominantly non-Christian region, the people of God were called to accomplish the church's mission together, except for those matters in which they could not participate in good conscience. The same theme was repeated in many regions and countries in the 1960s.

The concept of interfaith ministry is well established in American communities. Activities take the form of jointly sponsored lectures and seminars in theology and ministry, integrated curricula among theological seminaries, and events associated with special anniversaries and religious occasions. Groups of congregations, for example, resolve that what congregations can do together, they ought not to do alone. Religious bodies in local communities now routinely cooperate to address the plight of the homeless, develop food banks, and provide ministry in institutions too small to support a paid or full-time chaplain.

Such joint action is a witness to a common mission mandated by our identity as God's people. The people of God share the same life through worship and fellowship, care for each other, and employ God's gifts for the common good. As a corporate body and through its members God's people are called to continue the work of creation and redemption. One of the tasks, which is thereby mandated for us, is to care for all people, a task that is denoted by the Christian term, *pastoral care.*

Times of human crisis and rapid social change focus attention upon many human needs, but especially:

a. the need for community, because of the loneliness of people whose communities of origin reject them, and they become lost in a fragmented society;
b. the need for people to understand what is happening to them in the changing patterns of family and society, and in the struggles between competing values;
c. the need for human dignity, freedom, and justice in a society riddled with exploitation, racial and class discrimination, and political and economic injustices.

In such times as these, church and synagogue are called to participate in the continuing work of creation and redemption, so that there may be a clear and convincing sign of God's presence for people to see and follow. This is what is termed the *prophetic* function of God's people. The task of watching for and announcing the signs that God is present and active in the world was taken up at various times by the prophets, sung in the psalms, and prayed over by the devout in Israel (for example, see Ps. 130; Isa. 21:6 ff.; 52:8-10, 62:6-12; Jer. 4:16; 6:17; 31:6. Also Mark 13: 32 ff.; Luke 2: 25; 12:35 ff.). Two qualities are required to discern the way in which God is at work: "utter dependence upon God, a constant sensitive listening to [God] in [God's] Word and prayer, and a *thorough immersion in and identification with the suffering of the world*"[3] (our emphasis). Since most of us do not often meet these requirements because of our isolation from the world, our first task is to overcome this isolation. We are compelled by circumstances beyond our control—or, as believing people would say, by God—into a closer relationship with each other as the people of God. We are called to share the common resources of God in our ministries to people whose need is our call to service. As far as conscience and conviction allow, we should identify ourselves with all God's people and seek every means to demonstrate our unity.

Interfaith responses to the AIDS crisis almost invariably manifest this unity in local communities through hands-on services such as those of Houston's AIDS Care Teams, and through common worship that represents all who are engaged in ministry with people living with AIDS, both ministers and the people to whom that ministry is offered. Memorial services and services of healing and celebration are familiar settings for interfaith expressions of love and concern for people who have suffered the impact of AIDS. They express the united response of God's people on behalf of people who too often have felt compelled to suffer and grieve in secret. Families and friends who mourn the deaths of their loved ones are enabled to do so in worshiping communities in which they find acceptance and affirmation of their grief and of themselves. This may become the path along which they will find not only consolation but the renewal of joy and hope.

2. Maximizing the Community's Resources

The coordination of the activities of individual congregations by an interfaith council or network has proved an effective means of providing adequate and competent care to people who need and request it.

An interfaith network provides a basis for:

• coordination of education and care ministries in the community;

- maximizing the resources for AIDS ministries in the community;
- standardized training of Care Team members;
- coordination of Care Team activities with community agencies concerned with care for people living with AIDS;
- effective use of case management and referral skills and structures;
- coordinated presentation of the religious community's program to the wider community, and the development of local funding to support its ministries;
- provision for support and continuing education of team members and leaders;
- recruitment of additional Care Teams;
- access to clients;
- coordination of ministry activities with religious judicatories' plans and activities on local, state, and national levels;
- oversight of the program to ensure that it is non-judgmental and protects clients from religious proselytism.

Activities such as these help to form a foundation for the development of the community's response to HIV disease.

The following suggests the basic structures that can be established to achieve these objectives:

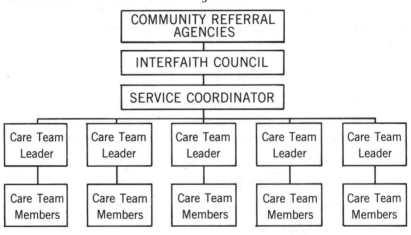

3. Interfaith AIDS Response as a Model for the Community

A. AIDS EDUCATION.

The nation has been reminded on many occasions by former Surgeon General C. Everett Koop, leading AIDS researchers, and the media that AIDS-awareness and risk-reduction education are our best weapons against the further spread of HIV. These efforts in local communities can be initiated effectively through coordinated community public health education programs, and congregations can constitute one of the most important components of such programs. Development of an interfaith response to AIDS calls for some form of network as an instrument of the respective congregations.

In many instances, the presentation of clergy seminars that provide current and accurate information concerning the AIDS crisis is a first step toward the recruitment of congregations to participate in the service, or Care Team, program. Such seminars should include basic medical information about means of infection, testing and counseling procedures, progression of HIV disease and related data; introduction to the psychosocial impact of HIV disease; issues related to spiritual support for people living with AIDS; and a description of the Care Team program as an appropriate channel for congregational ministry.

Clergy are encouraged to bring these matters to the attention of congregants, and to take the lead in providing appropriate AIDS awareness programs in their congregations. Such programs may be of greater effectiveness when sponsored by an interfaith group, such as a clergy alliance. Interfaith programs:

- make effective use of local educational resources and personnel;
- provide an effective witness to the wider community concerning the interfaith community's response to the threat of HIV and to people living with AIDS;
- develop a momentum leading to the development of an integrated, community-wide AIDS awareness and ministry program;

• assist in the shaping of policies with respect to county, city, school district, and indigent health care agencies regarding care for people living with AIDS.

B. CARE FOR PEOPLE LIVING WITH AIDS.

Service to the world is an essential calling of God's people. This is not a peripheral activity, but an aspect in the absence of which the claim to be the people of God is abrogated. We have to meet the needs of the world at the point where the world is feeling the greatest needs and encountering the greatest problems. Our motive springs from the knowledge of God's love for the whole of creation.

We deny our nature as the people of God if we fail to fulfill the servant role to which God calls us. This ministry is not offered from the ulterior motive of securing adherence to the faith stance of the care-giver. We pray that through the ministry of compassion offered by Care Team members, people whom we serve may experience the love God has for every creature; ministry is not a means to an end, but it is an end in itself. Yet it also stands as an expression to the secular society of our common humanity and the interdependence of the human community.

As a consequence to this commitment to service, it follows that the *quality* of the care offered to people living with AIDS is of paramount importance. The integrity of the Care Team program is directly dependent upon the integrity of the relationships individual members develop with their individual clients. This means, in turn, that the effectiveness of our work depends both on the adequacy of our team member training and the consistency of each member's participation in the process of supervision which, as we shall see, has been built into the system. These facets of the ministry are interdependent, and so are delineated in some detail in this book. We urge, therefore, that recruits considering a ministry to people living with AIDS should be advised of those expectations and challenged to commit themselves to a ministry of the highest order.

Goals of an Interfaith Program

1. To develop and maintain an AIDS interfaith network as a community of people who willingly serve others in accordance with their individual gifts, talents, and other personal and professional responsibilities.
2. To focus the attention of congregations and their communities on the needs of people living with AIDS, and develop service capabilities to meet those needs as a model for those communities.
3. To serve with other agencies in the development and provision of AIDS awareness programs for the respective age and cultural groups in the community.
4. To create and maintain a fellowship of mutual respect that will provide a context for understanding and will foster reconciliation between estranged people.
5. To provide a prophetic witness in communities facing the crisis evoked by the spread of HIV infection that will identify and redress injustices and gaps in community services related to people living with AIDS.
6. To present a positive response to oppression of people living with AIDS and encourage respect for them from individuals, agencies, and care-givers.

Methods

The primary service mode will be the development of congregationally-based AIDS Care Teams, consisting of members who:
1. Commit themselves to care for people living with AIDS;
2. Participate in training events to equip themselves for this ministry;
3. Are accountable to the Care Team leader and congregation;
4. Are committed to working cooperatively within the interfaith network, with the service coordinator, and with the other Care Teams;

5. Participate in regular supervision and continuing education opportunities.

The AIDS Interfaith Council participates with community health care agencies and other community-based organizations in coordinating AIDS service programs on behalf of people living with AIDS. It also provides AIDS education presentations to congregations and other community organizations.

The Interfaith Network

1. Administrative Functions

The interfaith network or council, as the organizational hub, is essential to the management of the program. The network represents the constituent congregations from which Care Teams are appointed, and plays an essential part in providing direction and management. It is expected to support fund-raising to meet program expenses, which may include:

- Administrative costs (clerical, phone, postage, travel, etc.);
- Provision for professional supervision of the program (see below);
- Employment of appropriate staff;
- Purchase of educational materials and team training packages;
- Training and continuing education events.

Some or all of these needs may be met without cost to the council. For example, administrative expenses may be carried by one or more of the congregations; patient care needs may be met from each congregation's customary relief funds; professional supervisory services may be provided on a voluntary basis by a Clinical Pastoral Education (CPE) supervisor or another appropriate professional (social worker or psychologist) as a contribution to the program. Office space and full- or part-time staff may be provided by participating congregations as in-kind contributions.

2. Relationship to the Local Community

The network promotes the Care Team ministry within the religious community, represents the ministry to the wider community, provides reports of the Care Teams' activities to religious bodies and to the public, and maintains communication with other community agencies, physicians, hospitals, governments, school district trustees, and so forth. The support of the program by the respective judicatories is critical to its effectiveness.

Reports of the teams' ministries are essential, since few programs survive without some acknowledgment that they play an important role that is respected and endorsed by their sponsoring bodies. For example, regular reporting by a Care Team to the congregation's board of deacons/elders keeps the attention of the congregation's members on the objectives of the Care Team program, namely, to minister to people living with HIV disease and to continue the education of the congregation regarding the impact of AIDS on the lives of its members. In turn, the program can have a ripple effect in the wider community. As citizens become aware of the ministry to people living with HIV disease, they may be better informed about the disease itself, and challenged by the examples of the congregations and their Care Teams.

As the interfaith council responds to growing numbers of people with AIDS, additional staff may be added and the council's structures expanded to provide more comprehensive services. For example, the AIDS Interfaith Council in Houston has developed a worship committee to plan and oversee the annual Sabbath Observance, a service of memorial and celebration, and other worship events; an advocacy committee that monitors state and county government response to the needs of people living with AIDS; and education, membership, and special events committees.

An expanded interfaith program structure might take the following form:

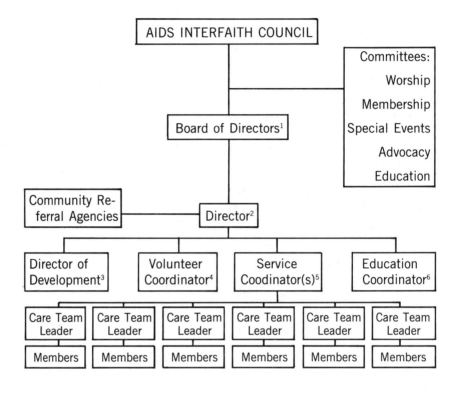

1. The administrative body may be a Committee, or, if incorporated, a board of directors or trustees.
2. The director (full- or part-time) is appointed by the Board to oversee the entire program. In smaller programs, the director and service coordinator functions may be centralized in one person. As the program grows, functions and responsibilities may be separated.
3. The director of development is the primary fund-raiser.
4. The volunteer coordinator responds to requests from congregations for information about the program, recruits new congregations, produces a program newsletter, etc.
5. One or more service coordinators fulfill the responsibilities outlined in the job description for this position (see below).
6. The education coordinator plans and facilitates AIDS education activities for Care Teams, local congregations, and community organizations.

3. Legal Liability

Volunteers and sponsors of a Care Team ministry properly may be concerned about legal liability. *It is imperative for sponsors of these ministries to research relevant state statute and case law to determine what provisions exist that bear upon volunteer functions.* It may be the case that sponsoring organizations and volunteers are immune from civil liability, provided certain conditions are met. However, such provisions vary from state to state.

For example, the Texas Charitable Immunity and Liability Act of 1987 grants immunity from civil liability to "a volunteer who is serving as a direct service volunteer of a charitable organization . . . for any act or omission resulting in death, damage, or injury if the volunteer was acting in good faith and in the course and scope of his duties or functions within the organization."[4]

The sponsoring organization of such charitable activities in Texas is granted limited liability, which can be covered by insurance. These exemptions from liability and limitations of liability do not apply to an act or an omission of a volunteer that is "intentional, willfully or wantonly negligent, or done with conscious indifference or reckless disregard for the safety of others."[5]

4. Leadership of the Program

Regardless of how carefully participating religious groups plan, and despite the best intentions with which the project is launched, ministry programs such as the one outlined here invariably founder unless the most meticulous attention is given to oversight of the day-by-day ministries of Care Team members. Leadership and supervision of the AIDS Care Team program is the keystone upon which the whole edifice stands or falls. Good intentions are not enough. The program director or service coordinator, supported by the interfaith council or committee, carries the primary responsibility of ensuring that congregational Care Teams are committed from the outset to be accountable for the effectiveness and quality of their work. We now turn to this aspect of the program.

NOTES

1. The terms *council* and *network* are used interchangeably in this document, reflecting common usage throughout the United States. Individual interfaith groups will make their own choice according to preference.
2. See, for example, Randy Shilts, *And the Band Played On* (New York: St. Martin's Press, 1987), p. 491.
3. J. Archie Hargraves, *Stop Pussyfooting Through a Revolution: Some Churches That Did* (New York: Stewardship Council of the United Church of Christ, 1965), p. 13.
4. The Texas Charitable Immunity and Liability Act, 1987.
5. Ibid.

CHAPTER THREE

Program Structure and Organization

Leadership and Oversight Functions

1. Importance of Strong Leadership

a. The success of any venture depends in large measure on the quality of its leadership. Service coordinators (see below) will facilitate effective ministry by Care Teams as they provide direction, structure, and consistent oversight of team leaders' activities.

b. The team leader's first task is the development of cohesion and direction within the team through the accustomed processes of good communication that develop group identity and facilitate bonding between members, regular meetings, starting and ending meetings on time, and other customary organizational tasks. Form and discipline are important aspects of the process. Inspiring members through precept and example are critical elements of leadership. A leader's modeling of team functions sets a pattern for team members. Leaders should not ask members to undertake tasks they have not assumed themselves.

2. Professional Supervision of the Program

a. Oversight, or supervision, is a basic leadership function. The model used in training and overseeing Care Teams is one derived initially from social work and employed by the religious community to equip clergy for pastoral ministry. Today, many laypeople enter supervised pastoral care training programs to learn or sharpen pastoral skills. "Clinical pastoral education" (CPE) is based on the simple reality that *learning by doing*, under the oversight of a person competent in the particular field, is the oldest and most time-honored method of education.

b. The AIDS Care Team program recognizes the importance of rigorous oversight at each level of the program. One means of ensuring competent oversight is to invite clinical pastoral supervisors to meet with the service coordinator and team leaders on a regular basis so that the team leaders' work is supervised, and in the process they may acquire supervisory skills as their own education is extended. CPE supervisors can be found in training centers in larger hospitals and mental health programs in most large cities. If CPE supervisors are not accessible, this service can be performed by pastoral counselors, clinical psychologists, or social workers with supervisory experience.

c. The supervisory process used in the Care Team ministry provides each team member with adequate support and ensures that the program's purposes are being implemented effectively; that is, that people with HIV disease are receiving caring and loving ministry.

d. The interfaith council, with a CPE supervisor or other professional as consultant, ensures accountability of Care Team ministries through supervision that is provided at each level of the program:

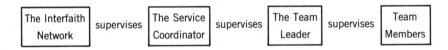

e. Each supervisor will be responsible for setting supervisory schedules in consultation with the service coordinator and team leaders. It is assumed that the supervisor's meetings with the service coordinator and team leaders should be held on a regular (usually monthly) basis, to provide consistent, intensive oversight and training of all participants.

Program Structure

1. The Service Coordinator

The service coordinator is the essential link between referral agencies, the Care Team program, and the people living with HIV disease for whom the teams care. In larger cities with comprehensive programs, the interfaith council may employ a director. If the council does not appoint a program director, the service coordinator serves as the "executive", or chief executive officer of the program. In smaller communities, the coordinator may be a pastor or other professional person whose congregation or agency incorporates this function in the individual's responsibilities. Alternatively, the position may be filled on a voluntary basis by a person who makes this role his or her commitment to ministry. In larger cities, the interfaith council may employ a coordinator.

The service coordinator plans and arranges training events, receives referrals from service agencies (e.g., hospitals, physicians, social workers), matches clients with Care Teams, and shares in the supervision of the program.

2. Job Description—The Service Coordinator

   a. oversees the scope and direction of spiritual ministry offered by team members to their clients;
   b. provides pastoral support to team leaders;
   c. receives inquiries from congregations interested in participating in the program, provides information and educational services regarding HIV disease and its impact on the community, recruits congregations, and advises on the selection of team members;
   d. designs and implements initial and continuing training programs;

e. schedules continuing report and leadership training sessions for team leaders;

f. reports to the interfaith council on teams' ministries;

g. in consultation with a professional supervisor, provides day-to-day oversight of the activities of team leaders and teams by:

  • establishing and maintaining a regular supervisory process;
  • maintaining contact with teams through regular visits;
  • assisting team leaders to resolve problems as they arise;

h. maintains regular contact with clients/patients to:

  • demonstrate the program's commitment to them and their families;
  • evaluate the quality and consistency of teams' activities;
  • receive reports regarding satisfaction/dissatisfaction with care, needs not met, etc.;
  • provide appropriate reports to social workers, physicians, and other referral sources, contributing to the effectiveness of the case management process.

Case Management

1. Clients are referred to the service coordinator by a variety of means. For example, requests may be made by:
     a. hospital social workers or discharge planners;
     b. AIDS service organizations;
     c. county or city health service agencies, physicians, etc.;
     d. individual referral (patient, family member, lover, or friend).

2. The service coordinator discusses with the client the type and extent of service requested. Some people find it

difficult to ask for help, acknowledge that help is needed, or accept it when offered. Some seek assistance only when their situations are desperate. Teams should be sensitive to the ambivalence that clients are likely to experience.

The referral process is known as *case management.* The term is widely used by social welfare agencies to refer to service coordination designed to ensure that each client is followed, so that no person is missed and particular needs are identified and served. Needs are met as they develop, facilitated by multi-directional communication. Team members receive assignments from the team leader and report activities to the team leader, who, in turn, keeps the service coordinator informed. The coordinator consults with the client and/or referral agency representatives as appropriate.

NOTE: Because many people living with HIV infection are compelled for a variety of reasons to have recourse to social welfare or charitable agencies, they are particularly vulnerable to any suggestion of "management" by people whose functions cast them in the roles of authority figures. The Care Team concept supports service coordination that respects and enhances patient autonomy. Care-givers must exercise care to avoid acting or giving the impression of acting in a parental manner. The integrity of the program depends on the sensitivity of each person in the chain of activities, as well as the level of accountability between the various components:

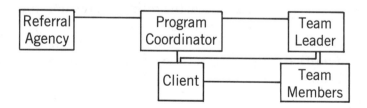

A case management network may be instituted by representatives of the community's agencies who meet regularly to review the case history of each person under care of the respective agencies and teams. Like all other community activities associated with the AIDS epidemic, this response is an effort to see that, as far as possible, the needs of each person living with AIDS are met. The involvement of the service coordinator provides liaison between health care agencies and the respective Care Teams.

Client Referral

1. Information about the Client

The following suggests the type of information sought by the service coordinator from the referral source, and provided to the Care Team leader:

a. **Personal:** Name, address, phone number, age, race. Most funding sources like to know the ethnic composition and the ages of the clients whom the ministry serves.

b. **Medical:** General description of the client's physical and mental status and level of need, including essential medical information, special conditions or infection control measures, insurance/social security, the name of the client's physician and the home nursing service if one is being used.

c. **Social:** When client is most likely to be home, other occupants in the residence, relationships with family members, and which, if any, family members are aware of the diagnosis.

d. **Identified Need:** Specific service (including frequency) requested.

This information may be prepared as a patient profile and made available to the team leader, who in turn provides it to assigned team members. However, this procedure should be accompanied by reminders of the client's right of privacy and confidentiality (see below). No action should be taken that renders the client vulnerable to needless or harmful exposure. (See appendix 2 for sample form).

2. *Procedure for Service Coordinator's Contact with Client*

   a. Client is referred to service coordinator by a social worker, discharge planner, other referral agent, or by self-referral. The coordinator will obtain the information identified above.

   b. The coordinator will phone or visit the client, confirm that the referring agency (social worker, physician, et al.) has reviewed the Care Team process with the client, and explain the terms and conditions of Care Team involvement.

   c. The coordinator should not promise that a team will be assigned (that is, do not say: "I have a team for you"), but that a team representative will be in touch with the client ("I will send someone to meet with you to discuss further your situation and determine whether we can respond to your needs").

   d. Referral of a client to a Care Team ideally will be made early in the course of the disease, when needs tend primarily to be for social contact and emotional support. Clients usually are referred to teams within the agreed geographic boundaries adopted by the team. If a client requests a team from a particular faith group, efforts may be made to link the client with a Care Team from that denomination. The client's wishes should be respected when possible.

3. *Procedure for Team's Contact with Client*

   a. The team leader or designated team members meet with the client within 48 hours of referral to assess needs and determine whether the team can accept the assignment. Location, the situation in the home, and so forth, may be reasons to decline the assignment.

b. During the introductory visit, the team leader/members confirm the level of perceived need, establish a "covenant" with the client, and clarify types and levels of commitments of both parties.

CAUTION: Team members should exercise care not to control the client; the client's identification of needs, rather than those of the visitor, should determine team members' responses.

Handling Referral Problems

1. *Problem*: When the introductory visit was made, it was determined that the client lived in a neighborhood that would be unsafe to visit at night. And there was unmistakable evidence or chemical substance abuse in the home.

   Response: The team members informed the team leader, who, in consultation with the service coordinator, decided not to accept the assignment.

   NOTE: It is not always possible to screen every element when referrals are made, but, as coordinators and team leaders become more familiar with the process, most of these situations may be avoided.

2. *Problem*: The referred client did not want the team's services; when the team leader phoned, the client declined help.

   Response: The team leader clarified the assistance the team could offer, and when it was declined, invited the client to phone the service coordinator if her situation changed and she desired a team's services.

3. *Problem*: The client's personality and the team's "personality," or that of the client and a particular team member, just did not match.

   Response: In the latter case, the team member may be reassigned to other clients. It should not be surprising that this may occur, and this possibility should be reviewed regularly with team members. When the *team* and a client just do not match, the issues should be reviewed carefully with the service coordinator; it may become an important learning situation for all concerned.

Client Confidentiality

Clients are vulnerable people. It is essential, therefore, to keep client information private. *Never* give information over the phone or in person to *anyone* without a legitimate right to know. For reasons of confidentiality, do not identify clients by name or address in written reports or newsletters.

On-Going Care Program

1. Escalating Needs and Demands

a. As a client's needs become more intense, additional team members may be assigned and/or the frequency of visits increased as appropriate. Note that, within reason, and depending on the availability of the team, the client should be encouraged to set the schedule. Excessive demands on the client's part should be referred to the leader for negotiation.

b. If the point is reached at which daily visits are indicated, the entire team may be used, so as to share the work load. NOTE: If the Care Team has developed intermittent care programs with a number of clients, and one person then requires intensive, daily support, the team leader should consult with the service coordinator. If warranted, the team may be relieved of some responsibilities so that the more intensive situation can be met, or additional team members may be recruited and trained. Team leaders should keep the service coordinator informed of emerging needs of their clients.

2. Client/Patient Financial Aid

The financial needs of some people living with AIDS may become catastrophic, and in any case, many are or will become indigent. Program personnel thus may face the question of whether to provide a fund from which to meet requests for financial aid. Service coordinators and team leaders should become familiar with community resources to meet clients' financial and material needs (e.g., Social Security, community welfare programs). Program leaders are advised to exercise caution in the establishment and management of a special client fund, and to establish guidelines for the *types* and *limits* of aid which will be provided, including limits on what one individual may receive.

NOTE: Care Teams are perceived as human resources, not social welfare or financial resources. We note, in the form of an "advisory," that the teams affiliated with the AIDS Interfaith Council in Houston, which originally developed programs to provide financial aid to their clients, now believe that is an unwise step, and have reversed the decision to offer direct financial assistance, except in cases of exceptional need.

THE CARE TEAM

Organization

1. Ideally, teams will have 14 to 20 members. Teams of this size:
   a. minimize commitment of individual members to a level that can be sustained over time;
   b. provide a solid base of mutual support and group maintenance;
   c. assist in the institution and consistency of accountability procedures;
   d. constitute an appropriate format for continuing education.

NOTE: A team may be started with 8 members. However, the team's activities will be limited until the number reaches 14 or more.

2. Team members will usually work in pairs. Pairing provides for:

a. support and consultation during visits;
b. reporting and accountability;
c. sharing of responsibilities during visits;
d. a greater degree of security, especially for evening or night visits.
e. healthier, more productive debriefing after visits.

If pairing rotates, team members should become more aware of each other's gifts and abilities, and bonding should be strengthened.

The Team Leader

1. *Job Description.* The team leader assumes responsibility for the management of the Care Team program on behalf of the congregation. The team leader:

a. receives referrals of clients from the service coordinator and assigns team members to the client(s);
b. contacts client following referral from service coordinator. While the first contact by the team leader may be by phone, followed by a home visit by two assigned team members, team leaders in some congregations have found that a personal visit by the leader, with subsequent follow-up visits, is effective in establishing a firm and mutually affirming relationship. This first visit may be used to establish expectations of both team members and client (see appendix 3);
b. convenes team meetings. (**NOTE**: The frequency of team meetings is determined by the team members. Meetings should be held at least bi-monthly, depending on the number of clients/patients under care, the intensity of their respective needs, and so forth; however, experience indicates monthly meetings are desirable);
c. supervises individual members;
d. coordinates team services;
e. keeps records of team members' ministries to clients and makes reports to service coordinator;

   f. in consultation with clergy staff, provides pastoral support
     to team members, with particular attention to grief
     ministry;

   g. ensures that adequate social, emotional, and spiritual
     support to meet relevant needs of members is incorporated
     in team activities;

   h. attends team leader continuing education activities:
- to keep abreast of HIV disease information;
- to acquire supervisory skills;
- to report team activities for supervision;
- to make suggestions for improvement of the program;
- to identify needs for additional education or training;

   i. reports to the congregation's clergy and administrative
     body on a regular basis.

2. *Periodic Changes of Leadership.* In this context, the team should ensure that the team leader receives adequate support from members and from the congregation. Most teams will find it beneficial to rotate team leadership at agreed points, e.g., after nine months or annually. It is important to anticipate this need, and to agree early in the life of the team on the format the team will follow.

The Team Member

1. *The Call to Minister.* Team members accept membership in the HIV Care Team as a ministry undertaken on behalf of the congregation. It is of the nature of religious congregations that membership entails participation in the congregation's life and mission, including its service functions. It is generally accepted that each member has a specific gift or capacity upon which the congregation can call in the meeting of its obligations. Not all members are gifted and called to the congregation's ministry to people living with HIV disease.

2. *Job Description.* The team member agrees:

a. to attend orientation and training sessions;
b. to provide an informed ministry of acceptance and support to people with HIV disease, their families, partners, lovers, and friends;
c. to fulfill accepted assignments by the team leader, unless renegotiated;
d. to keep the team leader informed regarding ministries with clients;
e. to attend team meetings for reporting and supervisory purposes;
f. to seek and accept supervision from the team leader and from other team members;
g. to contribute to the strengthening of team bonds through social and fellowship events;
h. to participate in continuing education events in a timely manner.

AN ADVISORY: Team members have found occasionally that their involvement in the Care Team program has been misunderstood by other people, e.g., relatives or neighbors. There have been occasional instances in which this involvement has met with negative responses. As with almost any concern, it is always easier to respond appropriately if one has anticipated these possibilities, and considered how they may be met. This is an important topic for individual and team reflection, particularly during the training of a new team, or the period of integration of new team members.

Team Member Communication

The provision of two-way communication between the service coordinator and team leaders helps to develop a sense of corporate identity, as well as ascertaining whether the needs of each person are being met. Similarly, since good communication plays such an important part in any team venture, special efforts to facilitate communication among team members will benefit the team's ministry. A "phone tree" that lists names and phone numbers of team members can be an effective tool of communication; each member in turn is responsible to contact two members, and each has easy access to others for information and support. The phone tree facilitates quick dispensing of essential information and enhances the bonding of team members, a vital aspect of peer care. A sample phone tree is illustrated here:

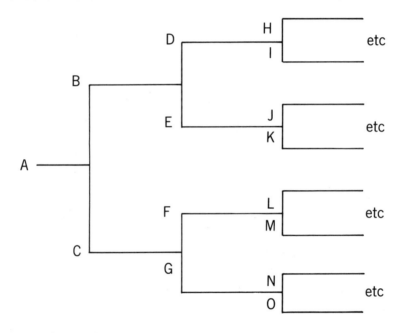

Contracting Team Services and Limitations

Teams affiliated with the AIDS Interfaith Council contract with clients during the intake interviews to provide such services as: social, emotional, and spiritual support; nutritional support (e.g., meal preparation), shopping, housekeeping tasks, transportation; assisting family members; and basic nursing care.

Terms and conditions:
  1. Each team is responsible for the content of its agreement with clients.

2. As teams increase their experience, many tend to modify their agreements with clients to reflect a client's status and needs, and the team's interests and experiences.
3. Teams are urged to be specific concerning each item. For example, what, if any, are the limits on "meal preparation," "transportation," or "assisting family members"?
4. The team's interests, and those of individual team members, will be best served if the services and any limits are written and left with the client.
5. Team members will need to use their discretion with respect to providing the client with their individual phone numbers. In general, the client will have the team leader's phone number, and may not need those of other members. In any case, a team member is free to provide a client with his or her own phone number, but not that of any other member unless permission has been given to do so.
6. Experience indicates that clients are appreciative of teams' ministries, and do not exploit or abuse this relationship. However, there may be occasions when a particular client, family, lover, or friend may be manipulative and make excessive demands on team members. These incidents should be reported to the team leader and brought to the attention of the entire team.

Integrating New Team Members

In the ordinary course of events, personal schedules and responsibilities of team members will change. Some members may withdraw from team activities, leading to the need to recruit and train new members. Training of new members may be undertaken by:

1. Inviting a potential recruit to meet with the team at regular meetings:
2. Pairing each new member with a more experienced team member during visits with clients;

(Steps 1 and 2, however, are preliminary actions until new recruits can attend an orientation/training session for a new team or for new recruits.)

3. Scheduling a team training session with the interfaith council staff, and/or including new team members in a network-wide training event incorporating a number of teams. Notices of training sessions should be sent to all team leaders, so that new members can be informed of training events.

Impact Upon Care Team Members of Ministry With People Living With Aids

Pastoral ministry of the intensity described in this book is demanding on the pastoral care-giver. Team members will find themselves experiencing the kinds and depths of feelings that they observe in patients and their families. They will face the same difficulties in letting go of clients with whom they have "bonded" over periods of months or years. Team members will also need to exercise self-discipline in their relationships with both clients and family members, for example, restraining tendencies to act in parental ways towards either. They will need to remain alert constantly to their own ambivalent responses of affection and irritation toward clients or family members.

To achieve these goals, careful structuring of the congregational Care Team program is necessary to provide an effective support system for team members. Members who are confident that they are accountable for their work through a process that ensures adequate oversight of each member will in turn make and keep their commitments to clients, be committed to the group process, and will capitalize on the learning opportunities afforded by participation in the program. These commitments, delineated in the following chapter, will then be reflected in compassionate and sensitive pastoral care.

CHAPTER FOUR

Team Member Commitments

Accountability

One of the prerequisites for appointment to the Care Team is commitment to full accountability for activities connected with the program. Because team members are representatives of their congregations' ministry and of the AIDS interfaith council, and are involved in direct person-to-person contact, it is essential that every member is subject to oversight and accepts the responsibility to report client visits.

The supervision of each person's work is an essential means by which to ensure "quality control" of the program, and to safeguard the interests of both the person receiving care and the care-giver. The secondary benefit of supervised ministry is the opportunity for improving care-giving skills through the shared learning entailed in supervision. As members report visits with clients, they learn to evaluate the effectiveness of their ministries, affirming what was done effectively and correcting less effective ministry.

Oversight is applied at each level of the program. Team leaders who supervise team members are themselves subject to oversight by the service coordinator, who is accountable to the interfaith council that sponsors the entire program. Since coordinators will be working closely with community agencies, they will be responsible to agency representatives for the quality of the Care Team program.

Service coordinators are also responsible to people living with AIDS whom, on behalf of Care Teams, they have agreed to serve. The entire program has only one goal: *to provide quality care to people adjusting to the impact of HIV disease.* Everything else is secondary to that goal, and justified only to the extent that people are receiving competent and sensitive care.

Commitment to Assigned Patients

Loyalty to people with HIV disease is as important as the expression of compassionate acceptance and ministry offered to them. It is important to remember that people living with HIV disease experience a series of losses and disappointments. People from whom they expected to receive support and understanding frequently abandon them. Patients may fear that physicians will cease to provide support, and, indeed, when patients' insurance benefits terminate, some do withdraw, leaving patients to depend on the public hospital system. Life may seem to be reduced to a series of physical, material, financial, emotional, and social losses. When this occurs, the Care Team's loyalty may be all that stands between a person with HIV disease and the overwhelming sense that no one cares. Much therefore depends upon team members' loyalty to patients. Before joining a team prospective members must determine their readiness to undertake the particular tasks to which the Care Team is committed and decide the level of participation they are able to make (see below). Once committed to this ministry of walking through the ordeal of HIV disease with clients and their loved ones, such loyalty can become a source of strength and comfort. Such fidelity can be a manifestation of the fidelity of God's love toward people living with HIV disease.

Openness to Personal and Pastoral Growth

When one opens oneself to pastoral ministry with another person, the result is a process in which, in this living relationship, the care-giver finds that openness exposes both parties, the care-giver and the receiver of care, to growth. Pastoral theologian Jasper Keith reminds people called to pastoral ministry that, if they are really to be available and to listen to people in crisis, they must first be able to listen to themselves. Keith notes, "inextricably bound to my ability to listen to me is my sense of self-value and self-acceptance. For me to listen to me is for me to engage the most threatening aspect of my being."[1] He adds that such openness to whatever comes may be anxiety-provoking, and more often than not we resist such experiences of anxiety.

For example, to be present with someone who is critically ill, and perhaps near death, means that care-givers must be open to their fears of illness and death. In the course of our daily lives, most of us avoid confronting issues of mortality. We prefer not to be reminded of our finitude. When ministering to a person with terminal HIV disease, there are few hiding places, and we come face to face with some of our deepest fears.

AIDS researchers have documented the burdens placed upon care-givers who devote themselves to care for people living with AIDS, and the need to establish personal support systems for care-givers who continue to see their best efforts seemingly defeated by "this dreadful scourge."[2] Paul Volberding, a San Francisco physician who has been caring for people with AIDS since 1982, notes that AIDS poses "severe and chronic stress" for the care-giver, and individuals and teams who care for people living with AIDS must be provided with resources to alleviate these stresses.[3] If unrelieved, for example, such stresses may be manifested in irritability among Care Team members, which will impede team relationships and supervision, or in impaired relationships between members and their clients, which may result in less effective and compassionate ministry. Thus, support for the care-givers is an important aspect of Care Team life (see below).

It is difficult to imagine any person engaging in the intense activities and relationships that characterize care for people living with AIDS without being compelled to reflect on the meaning of events and interactions for the care-giver's own personal development. Thus, when trusting relationships are established between clients and team members, care-givers are in the privileged position of being welcomed into another person's life at a vulnerable and perhaps lonely time. Patients struggle with the desire to preserve their autonomy, yet are aware of their need to reach for and accept help. In this setting, care-givers may enter new worlds of self-understanding and personal growth.

Similarly, if the care-giver is a person of faith, this privileged position offers a further possibility. As the two people are present to each other, ultimate issues may assume spiritual dimensions, and the team member's "pastoral identity" may be shaped and strengthened. Keith suggests that the writers of scripture, recording their understanding of creation, were not asking deep, theoretical questions about their origins, about "being." Rather, "they were asking about their ultimate security in a most frightening world," and exploring the meaning of their existence in relationship to other human beings. They searched for faithful answers and healing solutions to human struggles.[4]

It is into this adventure, with its potential and challenges for self-understanding and self-growth that Care Team members enter when pressing the door-bell at a home that has been invaded by HIV disease.

Commitment to the Group Process and the Care Team

Among the "tasks" entailed in the caring process, none is more arduous or demanding than the "work" of grieving. Because we minister to people facing a disease for which there is still no known cure, Care Team members often sit with patients in end-stage AIDS. One of the promises teams have made to people living with HIV disease is that they will not die alone. None of us imagines it is easy, or comfortable, to undertake the most intimate tasks of ministry outlined above. The reality of catastrophic illness and the nearness of death bring added pain. Team members know, as they accept responsibility for the care of a new client, that they may expect to share in his or her death.

These realities, together with the necessity to monitor the quality of team care, make it essential that the integrity of the Care Team itself be maintained and protected. This is a task in which every team member shares. Commitment to this group process is a manifestation of the commitment to the patients themselves. Group maintenance, or group building, therefore, is essential to compassionate ministry to people living with AIDS, since it determines the quality of group members' relationships to each other and to clients.

Group Building

The process of group building and group maintenance provides the resources by which members are prepared for their various activities. The means by which teams accomplish these goals vary widely. They may include the following features:

1. Regular report sessions when individual members present an account of their activities. The team leader usually facilitates this process, which encompasses any problems that have arisen in relationships to a particular client or patient, new concerns that have not previously been encountered, and administrative matters, such as schedule changes.

2. Some teams restrict their meetings to administrative matters, such as schedule changes. Other teams use the opportunity for social events linked to the team's ministries. The evening may begin with a covered dish meal and include non-structured time for fellowship and companionship.

Clients may be invited to some sessions, both to meet all the group members and to assist in meeting clients' needs for socialization. The presence of clients/patients also enables the group to receive direct feed-back from people who receive its ministries.

CAUTION:Whether clients are present or not for social events, teams ought to meet in supervisory sessions in which members report their visits with clients for oversight and continuing learning. These supervisory sessions should be restricted to team members.

3. The evening may include a time for reflection, during which relationships with patients who have since died are remembered and treasured and grief ministry to colleagues effected.

4. In cities in which a number of teams work cooperatively, the interfaith network may arrange functions at which the groups meet together for purposes of communication concerning the community-wide response to AIDS, AIDS-information updates, continuing education opportunities, socializing, and so forth.

5. In cases in which members of one team become knowledgeable concerning specific aspects of AIDS (for example, relationship to substance abuse, county/state welfare systems, Social Security benefits, legal issues, etc.), these resources can be identified and shared through continuing education programs designed for individual teams or groups of teams.

Pastoral Care: A Ministry of Listening

Elisabeth Kübler-Ross was complimented during a television interview on her remarkable contribution to our understanding of human grief. She responded modestly that, although she is a physician, she had never "healed" anyone, nor found a cure for a disease; all she had done was to sit and listen to people, and *hear* them.

When writing or talking about *listening* to people, and *hearing* them, one wants to emphasize these words by qualifying them, and talk instead about *really* listening, and *really* hearing! Too often, we half-listen, waiting for the other person to end what he or she is saying so that we can take over the conversation. When I "half-listen," I am signaling not only that what the other is saying is of lesser importance than what I have to say, but that I am less concerned for him or her than for myself.

When the intent of a visit is pastoral, and not merely social, the care with which we listen will determine the quality of the pastoral relationship. From this perspective, listening is a demanding process that requires a high level of commitment on our part. *Real* listening is hard work.

1. "Half-Listening"

One of the reasons we tend to half-listen is our preoccupation with assuming responsibility for other people's problems, with the accompanying implication that we know best what they ought to do, and are ready to announce our solutions! We must be able to sit with the people for whom we care, disciplined by the knowledge that the responsibility for resolving issues and problems must remain with them. The most we can offer in many situations is help in identifying and exploring options that may be open to clients.

2. Listening to Feelings

It is important to listen to the *facts*, or the information, that the other person is sharing with us. It is even more important to listen to the *feelings* the person is expressing. Pieces of the story—the facts—are the vehicles that convey how the other person feels about what he or she is facing. *Empathy* is the term for this quality of listening. It means that one is open to the other person's pain and ready to enter into that pain, to the extent one person can ever enter another's world. It means, equally, being a part of the other person's joys and moments of celebration. (Too often, we think of pastoral care only in terms of pain and suffering; joy and celebration are also part of ministry). It is important, however, to distinguish between *care* and *counseling*. Care Teams offer care, stopping short of counseling.

3. Distinguishing Between "Care" and "Counseling"

The distinction between pastoral *care* and pastoral *counseling* must always be preserved. *Pastoral care* refers to the general ministry of care that each religious community provides to its members, and to the wider community in appropriate circumstances (for example, at times of local or national suffering or crisis). *Pastoral counseling* applies to the professional function of personal or family counseling or psychotherapy provided by people who are licensed (e.g., clergy, social workers, psychologists or psychiatrists) to provide this service. Care Team members' activities (unless the member is professionally qualified) are limited to the general area of pastoral care. Counseling needs, when identified, should be referred to the team leader for appropriate referral to a qualified counselor.

Lay ministers may recognize the opportunity or need for counseling and suggest means of obtaining this assistance. Many clergy have at least some training in this field and will be familiar with counseling services in the community. Congregations may play an important role by supplementing their Care Teams services with emotional and grief support groups, or even facilitate the provision of group therapy services related to the needs of people living with HIV disease: client/patient, family members, lovers, and others.

Pastoral care for people living with HIV disease may include ministry to people in crisis, and, almost always, to people in grief.

4. RESPONSE TO CRISES

Ventures into counseling and problem solving should be undertaken, if at all, only in consultation with the team leader. However, because people living with AIDS are confronted with continuing crises, often of growing intensity, the care-giver's ministry will inevitably involve helping the person deal with emergencies. While keeping in mind the limitations sketched above, team members will often be asked by the client/patient to participate at very basic levels of decision-making. It is of the essence of pastoral care that, while ready to explore options, or to help clarify and sort through issues, the responsibility for choice must always remain with the other person, that is, the client (or family member, lover, or designated proxy). In most instances, common sense will suggest the form ministry may take. For example:

Client, in panic: I don't know what to do. I am so afraid.

Team Member: I can see that you are upset, and can feel something of how scary it is for you. It seems you are up against a wall, with nowhere to go. . . .
(Later)

Team Member: I'm glad I can be here with you. Let's look together for some options. For example, have you thought about . . .

Remember, too, that there will be times when feelings will be so intense that you are, literally, at a loss for words. Learn to be comfortable with your own feelings of helplessness:

Team Member: I don't know what to say. I feel helpless. The best I have to offer is just being here.

At such moments, silence may be your most appropriate and meaningful response. Some other possible responses:

- That is something I cannot answer. If it is OK, I'll ask (our team leader) to help with that.
- I can see that what (he/she) said made you angry.
- That is some comfort. But you still have to face . . .
- You must have all sorts of mixed feelings about that.
- I like the way you dealt with that.
- What can I do that will be the greatest help?
- That is beyond my ability; I don't have that level of training. But I think I can put you in touch with someone who can help you with it.

5. Response to Grief

Grief ministry is at the heart of care for people living with AIDS. The inseparability of grief from progressive HIV disease forces both client/patient and care-giver to begin the work of grieving early in the relationship. The fear that one is HIV positive carries with it the dread of learning that it is a reality. The often protracted period of wondering when symptoms will appear likewise is darkened with anticipatory grief. The first appearance of *Pneumocystis carinii* pneumonia (PCP) or Kaposi's sarcoma (KS) or other opportunistic infections may be accompanied by premonitions of death. Recurrences and intensification of symptoms may serve to heighten the grief.

Throughout this time, perhaps extending over many years, there are frequent periods when the patient feels well, is able to continue employment, and is buoyed by the news of the latest promising medical discovery. Hope is reborn and all seems right with the world. But just as often, disappointments arise like thunderclouds to blot out the light. These are testing times for both patient and care-giver, darkened by the realization that people living with AIDS are, in the main, newborns, adolescents, or adults facing death much too prematurely.

Care-givers are learning that, in the course of ministering to people living with AIDS, they are walking with patients who are confronted with the reality of their mortality, and at the same time must come to terms with the meaning of that reality for themselves.

Researchers in the social sciences suggest that people facing terminal illnesses seem to experience three characteristic responses:

- Shock, numbness, and disbelief;
- Anger, sadness (depression), and/or other grief responses;
- A measure of resolution, or "acceptance," characterized by a variety of responses, including resignation, denial, hope for a cure, or, alternately, a positive attitude that life will be lived at its fullest, however long or short.

The care-giver, therefore, must be constantly alert to this pervasive grief, closer to the surface at some times than at others, but always taxing to emotional and spiritual strength, and prone to erode whatever determination the patient has gathered to oppose the threatening infection. This is all the more critical in light of research which shows that when loss of control over vital life forces and decisions is experienced, the immune system is apt to be further weakened.[5]

In this context, pastoral ministry to people living with AIDS is essentially grief ministry that both attends to the manifestations of grief and supports an acceptance of reality of which hope should be a mainstay. It is this message, mingling compassion and hope, that is the central focus of the love Care Team members express to people living with HIV disease through their daily ministrations.

Care for the Care-Givers

Such a ministry, however, is possible only if care-givers are in touch with their own mortality, as well as being aware of the impact of anticipated death upon patients. Team members will confront this threat, directly or indirectly, with each crisis in patients' lives, for example,

- with changes in health status;
- if the patient or family member initiates discussion of death, its inevitability, or its meaning;
- when questions are raised about the meaning of life, especially when it is fore-shortened;
- if the patient initiates discussion of his/her funeral service, requests the team member's help in writing the service, invites the team member to participate in the service, or to mediate with the patient's family concerning such desires.

An effective way to work through these concerns is to discuss them openly at team meetings. Grief can become immobilizing when it is unrecognized, and therefore is likely to remain unresolved. If not brought to resolution, grief is likely to "pile up," until it has reached dimensions that can incapacitate the care-giver.

Care Teams in the Houston interfaith council, which have ministered to over 500 people with AIDS since 1986, of whom over 350 have died, are witnesses to the wisdom and necessity of working through the grief of team members as a group function. Team members:

- accept responsibility for one another;
- are alert to indicators that the team or one its members has grief work to do;
- share in memorial services following the death of a patient;
- periodically reflect on what each patient has meant to members, reflections that may be accompanied by both tears and hilarity.

The task of caring for each care-giver in the Care Team network is a joint responsibility that is met fully only when shared by every participant in the program.

Understanding the Needs of People Living With Aids

Just as it is essential to build the AIDS Care Team ministry around appropriate structures to ensure accountability through consistent oversight and provisions for continuing education of team members, it is also incumbent upon each participant to strive to understand the emotional and spiritual anguish encountered by people living with AIDS. It is never appropriate for a caring person to say to another individual, "I know *just* how you feel." Yet care-givers must take a risk, namely, to place themselves in places and positions where they are vulnerable to the hurts and pains of the people for whom they care.[6] The pain that the other person is feeling will wash, like a wave, over one's self, as one enters the other's world.

Not, of course, that one can ever enter fully into another person's life. But to the extent that this privilege is granted by people living with AIDS to Care Team members, we do well to remember to take off our shoes, for we walk on holy ground. To do so, we need to know something of the psychosocial factors that affect both people living with AIDS and care-givers. These concerns are addressed in the next chapter.

NOTES

1. Jasper N. Keith, Jr., "Healing in Theological Perspective," *The Pastor as Counselor*, Earl E. Shelp and Ronald H. Sunderland, eds. (New York: The Pilgrim Press, 1990).
2. Paul Volberding, "Supporting the Health Care Team in Caring for Patients with AIDS," *Journal of the American Medical Association* 261 (February 3, 1989), 747-48.
3. Ibid.
4. Keith, "Healing in Theological Perspective."
5. See, for example, Silvano Arieti, *The Intrapsychic Self* (New York: Basic Books, 1967), p. 73; Jerry M. Burger, "Desire for Control, Locus of Control, and Proneness to Depression," *Journal of Personality* 52: 1 (March, 1984), 71-89; and Judith Rodin, "Aging and Health: Effects of the Sense of Control," *Science* 233 (September 19, 1986), 1271-1276. For data regarding the relationship between stress, bereavement, and depression and immunocompetence, see Joseph R. Calabrese, Mitchel A. Kling and Philip W. Gold, "Alterations in Immunocompetence During Stress, Bereavement, and Depression: Focus on Neuroendocrine Regulation," *The American Journal of Psychiatry* 144 (September, 1987), 1123-1134.
6. See, for example, Earl E. Shelp and Ronald H. Sunderland, *AIDS and the Church* (Philadelphia: The Westminster Press, 1987), chs. 3 and 4; also Samuel E. Karff, "Ministry in Judaism: Reflections on Suffering and Caring," *A Biblical Basis for Ministry*, Earl E. Shelp and Ronald H. Sunderland, eds. (Philadelphia: The Westminster Press, 1981), ch. 1; and Klaus Seybold and Ulrich B. Mueller, *Sickness and Healing* (Nashville: Abingdon Press, 1981).

CHAPTER FIVE

Psychosocial Needs of People Living With AIDS

An understanding of psychosocial factors associated with HIV disease is essential to the design of AIDS awareness and risk-reduction education and to the development of service programs to meet the needs of people living with HIV disease. The predominant factors include the demographics of the epidemic in the area (city, county, state), modes of HIV transmission, the level of stigma attached to HIV infection, and the intensity of anguish experienced by people living with HIV disease.

AIDS is still regarded by many people in the United States as a disease that primarily affects homosexual white men. While it remains true that male-to-male sexual contact represents the most common route of HIV transmission (approximately 61 percent of the cumulative total[1]), it is more accurate to describe AIDS as an infectious disease that can be transmitted sexually, that is, by either homosexual or heterosexual contact. It can also be transmitted by common use of contaminated needles and syringes, or by a pregnant woman to her fetus. In New York and other eastern cities, the number of new cases among intravenous drug users and their sexual partners now exceeds new cases among gay men.

As of December 1989, over 42 percent of all cases of AIDS

occur in people of color, yet these groups comprise approximately 19 percent of the population. Of the cases reported between June 1981 and January 1988, the Centers for Disease Control (CDC) report that the incidence of AIDS among white adults in the United States is 432 per million, while for blacks it is 1,223 per million and for Hispanics 1,179 per million.[2]

With respect to communities of color in the United States, women are more statistically at risk than males; black and Hispanic women account for 71 percent of all women with AIDS.[3] Of children under the age of 13 years diagnosed with AIDS in the United States through October 1989, 421 are white; 1,006 are black; and 462 Hispanic.[4]

AIDS may thus be described as a disease of the disadvantaged, the marginalized, and the disenfranchised.[5] As a consequence, HIV-infected people are not only stigmatized but frequently are ostracized by friends, and may be alienated from their families. Such negative responses to people with AIDS are probably due to persistent, widespread ignorance of the disease and its demographics. Despite continuing efforts to educate the general public concerning modes of transmission, for example, Foundation for Interfaith Research and Ministry staff receive a steady stream of inquiries concerning the possibility of infection from kissing, use of common bathroom space, and the need for sterilization of household items used by people with AIDS.

Continuing tolerance of discrimination against people with AIDS, however, is a consequence of the general public's perception of the people who constitute the majority of people infected by HIV. Because HIV disease is striking people of color, drug users and their sexual partners, and gay men with special severity, these communities are doubly vulnerable. They are people who often experience themselves as devalued and oppressed, despite civil rights victories since the 1960s. They are at a higher statistical risk for infection, and, if infected, more likely to progress to AIDS. They then face a future darkened by the prospect that HIV disease, given current therapeutics, may prove to be 100 percent fatal. More immediate threats, namely, possible loss of employment, loss of health insurance, and the daily anxiety that they may be ostracized by people in their communities further undermine their security.

HIV disease, however, is not restricted to these marginalized groups. Any person who comes into contact with the virus may be infected. For example, heterosexual adults and adolescents may risk HIV infection through sexual intercourse with an HIV-infected partner. In such cases, for example, the risk of transmission by infected men to their spouses and to newborns is real. There is growing evidence from communities ranging from major cities to small rural towns[6] that Care Team members increasingly may be ministering to families in which husband, wife, and child are HIV positive or have been diagnosed with AIDS.

These issues become concerns for team members in relationships with clients who are struggling with feelings of guilt, shame, and anger. As we point out in subsequent sections, the appropriate response is one of listening to expressions of grief, manifested in feelings of hurt, confusion, anger, and, perhaps, betrayal and despair. For the team member, the source of infection ought not be an issue, since our concern is not *how* clients or patients became HIV-infected, only that they are ill and their sickness is a claim upon our care and compassion.

One of the few consolations now emerging is the fact that people with AIDS are living longer, probably because of earlier detection and earlier intervention with more effective treatment modalities. Nevertheless, people living with HIV disease often live fear-filled lives, lack adequate support systems, and, to meet basic needs of shelter, food, companionship, and other daily requirements may be forced into dependency upon such services and ministries as those offered by AIDS Care Teams. Loss of control is itself a burden and a threat. Loss of independence may be a source of anger and depression, and stress or perceived loss of control has been shown to further weaken the body's immune response just at the time when a well-functioning immune system is vital to the person's health (see note 5, ch. 4). This is one of the grave threats faced by all seropositive people (that is, people whose blood tests are positive for antibodies to HIV), including hemophilia and coagulation-disorder patients who have acquired HIV infection.

Hemophilia Patients

Between January 1981 and December 1989, over 1,000 cases of hemophilia-associated HIV disease have been reported to the Centers for Disease Control.[7] Nearly 92 percent of people with severe hemophilia A in the United States have been exposed to HIV disease.[8] AIDS is now the primary cause of death among hemophiliacs, "surpassing hemorrhage and liver disease, previously the leading causes in this population."[9] AIDS has had a devastating impact upon the 150,000 to 230,000 Americans with hemophilia. Most people who have this hereditary blood clotting disorder rely on regular infusions of blood plasma products, some of which were contaminated by HIV and distributed prior to the development of HIV screening methods in 1985.

Hemophilia patients with AIDS face many of the same emotional stresses and anxieties as other AIDS patients, but in addition, are confronted with factors peculiar to this patient group. First, in common with people who acquired AIDS through blood transfusions, they often feel and are often described as "innocent parties." Their infection is traced to their dependence on the use of blood products as life-saving treatment modalities. Second, many hemophilia patients who, in many cases since childhood, have depended upon the medical profession for their very lives now feel betrayed by the medical community. A loss of faith has been noted, not only in blood products (despite the fact that, since 1985, the concentrates are virtually free of virus) but in the medical and scientific communities in general. HIV infection also has compounded the difficulty of adjusting to being hemophilic, leading to isolation, dependency on the family, anger at the medical system, and fear of disclosure of hemophilia and HIV infection.[10]

The consequence of this loss of trust is often outrage toward physicians, which is exacerbated by rage toward the people who now may be "blamed" for their infection, namely, drug users and gay men. Fear and anger often are deepened further because many hemophilia patients are afraid they may have endangered sexual partners, or must face the realization that they have already unknowingly transmitted the infection not only to spouses but to their children. The level of trauma for hemophiliacs whose use of blood products began prior to 1985 is so high that many patients have refused to participate in HIV testing, while others who have submitted to testing have declined to learn the results. Many patients keep their infection secret from family members and close friends, erecting additional barriers that may intensify isolation when support is most needed.

Team members may be confronted with different concerns, depending on the ages of hemophilia patients. Some HIV antibody positive men with hemophilia may have excluded their sexual partners from general education concerning the risk of HIV infection associated with treatment for hemophilia, and wives may be in danger if their sole source of information about AIDS is "filtered through their husbands' determined mental set to 'beat the odds' or downplay the risks."[11] Some couples seem to remain willing to risk HIV infection to the spouse or fetus. Care-givers should avoid passing judgment on such couples and alienating them from available resources.[12] The care-giver must be able to maintain a pastoral relationship characterized by responding to expressions of anger with patience and by sensitive listening to anxiety, guilt, or other manifestations of the burden of illness.

Adolescents with hemophilia, like all teenagers, are faced with issues of independence, peer acceptance, and self-esteem. These tasks tend to be more difficult for HIV-seropositive hemophilic adolescents who are coping with a chronic disease at the time when they are attempting to resolve personal concerns of sexual identity and mortality. Although most health care personnel believe children should be told of their HIV status, parents of teenage children may have restricted information concerning HIV infection from reaching them.[13] Team members must exercise care not to contravene parental decisions. A survey of parents of hemophiliac children indicates high levels of anxiety, which in turn can reinforce the tendency toward overprotective parenting, as well as impairing healthy intimacy between parents and children.[14]

Pastoral care for hemophilia patients who have contracted AIDS may take the form of listening to expressions of helplessness, rage, and grief. Since the care-giver cannot alter the fact or the means of infection, listening to patients' accounts of their torment and grief may be supplemented by assisting their exploration of those options which are open to them. These may include identifying areas in their lives over which they can choose to exercise control, serving as sources of strength and support to other family members, and following through with the decision to live their lives to their fullest abilities. One of the care-giver's more important roles may be encouraging patients or their parents to continue with appropriate medical appointments and treatments, and to find other avenues through which to resolve anger and the fear of disclosure.

People Living With Blood Transfusion-Related AIDS

Some people unknowingly contracted HIV infection through blood transfusions prior to the development of HIV screening methods in 1985. Since the virus may not produce symptoms for ten years or longer, some people infected via this mode of transmission may develop symptoms of HIV disease as late as 1995, and perhaps longer. Further, although screening for HIV contamination is now routine, blood banks acknowledge that it is not yet possible to claim that the blood supply is entirely safe. Thus, a small number of people receiving blood transfusions may continue to be infected during the 1990s.[15] This will remain a source of anxiety in the general public, and a continuing concern for health care personnel.

People thus infected may experience stresses similar to those faced by other people living with AIDS. Withdrawal from family and social relationships, anxiety, distrust of medical and scientific professionals, and anger due to perceived injustice are typical reactions. Depressive symptoms may include sadness, helplessness, hopelessness, lowered self-esteem, suicidal thoughts, and anticipatory grief.

Like people with hemophilia-related AIDS, these people often experience rage toward the individuals and groups of people whose behaviors, however unknowingly, contributed to the presence and spread of HIV infection in society. They may perceive themselves as "victimized" through no fault of their own and experience real or imagined stigmatization from acquaintances, family members, and their communities. Anger may be vented toward family members or friends with an intensity that further alienates them from their customary sources of emotional and spiritual support. Care-givers' acceptance of outbursts of feelings, patience in listening to them, and encouragement to maintain and enhance life-styles and options will play an important part in enabling these clients to cope with their situations.

Drug Users With AIDS

The relationship of AIDS and drug use raises critical pastoral and moral concerns for Care Team members and their congregations. Intravenous drug users (IVDUs) are susceptible to HIV infection through the sharing of hypodermic needles and syringes. The CDC reports that by November 1989, twenty-six percent of AIDS cases were due to factors directly related to IV drug use, an increase of two percent over the previous year. Fifty-three percent of HIV infection in black AIDS patients and fifty-six percent in Hispanic patients is attributable to infection through IV drug use.[16] While the drug "crack" is not taken intravenously, it is reported that crack use is usually accompanied with heightened sexual activity, which may lead to HIV transmission, as in the case of IVDUs, to sexual partners of child-bearing age. As a result, the number of neonates with AIDS is increasing rapidly; the rate of increase in 1989 was approximately 12 percent.[17]

Teams caring for drug users with AIDS report high levels of frustration and irritation with some clients. While we have noted that, following consultation with the program coordinator, a team appropriately may ask to be relieved of a client's care, this action may be accompanied by a feeling on the team's part that the team has "given up" or failed, perhaps leading to disillusionment and guilt, and a decision to decline assistance to other drug users with AIDS.

There is little doubt that this patient population is likely to try the patience of team members. For example, drug or alcohol use can affect a person's decision to adopt consistent AIDS risk-reduction behaviors. Since drug use poses a threat to the body's immune response, a drug user who becomes infected with HIV often faces the virus with a compromised immune system, may be more prone to a wide spectrum of opportunistic or other infections, and progression to AIDS is likely to be rapid and overwhelming.

Care-givers may regard drug use as irresponsible weakness on the part of clients, whose perceived lack of self-discipline and "moral" behavior may tempt Care Team members to withdraw support. The following perceptions by care-givers may reinforce these concerns:

a. *Drug use is a weakness.* However, many researchers hold that substance abuse is a chronic, progressive disease that is treatable.

b. *Substance abusers can be highly manipulative, using aggression, flattery, and verbal intimidation to dominate care-givers.* Anger, blame, or guilt, which may be experienced by Care Team members, should not be used to control drug users, but should be acknowledged and processed as part of the team's supervisory functions.

Team members need to be aware constantly that the presentation of such concerns for supervision is essential not only to protect the integrity of the relationship with the client, but to enhance the well-being and learning of both client and care-giver.

c. *Drug users have no one but themselves to blame for their health status.* While it may be true that IVDUs have engaged in risk behaviors that resulted in HIV infection, resort to chemical substance abuse cannot be assigned simplistically to "moral weakness." It is often influenced by factors that can be traced to family and societal environments, and behaviors that society has implicitly sanctioned or condoned.[18]

The crisis of HIV infection may accentuate the destructive effects of drug use behaviors. In common with other groups of patients who are HIV positive or have been diagnosed with AIDS, drug users may enter the health care system in intense psychological distress (see ch. 5 below). In a life-threatening situation, they must cope with anxieties related to dying and death, regret evoked by awareness of previous behaviors, and the consequences of substance withdrawal. In order to be able to meet the physical, psychosocial, and spiritual needs of drug users with AIDS, Care Teams should seek the professional counsel and support of mental health personnel who are familiar with drug counseling.

Care Team Ministry with Drug Users

What attitudes should Care Team members adopt toward substance abusers with AIDS?

First, care-givers should attempt to assess the extent and effects of substance use, clients' awareness of their problems, and their readiness to accept the Care Team's agreement for service. Care Teams are entitled to determine whether they can accept clients, or continue their care if the clients refuse to make a good-faith effort to respond to the opportunities offered by the team.

Second, the Care Team leader should ensure that guidelines are established that delineate the specific obligations of the team and the client/patient.

Third, since denial usually accompanies the onset of a life-threatening illness, and subsides only as the person accepts the reality of the crisis, the combination of HIV infection and substance addiction may create unusual problems for the care-giver. Substance abusers regularly resort to denial as a primary

PSYCHOSOCIAL NEEDS 79

defense against acknowledging their problems and the effects of addiction. It is appropriate for team members to inform a client that they are aware of the drug use and to challenge the client's denial. Open, frank discussion of the implications of AIDS and drug use will help to avoid deception and ambiguous communication.

Fourth, as indicated above, this area of Care Teams' responsibilities should receive careful attention. Service coordinators are advised to consult with substance abuse and other community-based agencies in order to provide continuing education opportunities to Care Teams and to ensure coordination of resources to assist drug-use-related AIDS clients.

Pastoral concerns include the Care Team members' capacity to offer acceptance to substance abuse clients without compromising either accepted mental health guidelines or their own values and commitments to quality support of clients. Team members should offer their care and support activities with the explicit understanding between members and clients that clients will be held responsible for their actions. Care Team members should keep team leaders and other Care Team members informed of the nature and extent of their relationships with clients; there can be no secrets within teams concerning client behaviors. Because substance abusers tend to be particularly adept at manipulating care-givers, it is especially important that members work consistently in pairs, and that they submit reports of their ministry with drug users for supervision.

Ministry With Pediatric AIDS Patients and Their Families[19]

The rising incidence of HIV infection in newborns corresponds to the increasing rate of HIV infection among women of child-bearing age. This vertical transmission of HIV adds another dimension to AIDS ministries. Many Care Teams will be called upon to serve families with AIDS in which one or more children are infected or symptomatic, having been infected by the mother prior to or during birth. The mother's route of infection will be traceable to one of the established modes of transmission, and her husband or partner also may be infected.

These situations present significant challenges to care-givers, whose work will involve relating to both children and adults who present a variety of needs related to their physical, social, financial, and emotional states. These needs will be further intensified if IV drug use or other substance abuse is a factor.

With few exceptions, Care Teams assigned to a pediatric AIDS patient will be called upon to minister to the family unit, however configured. Separation of a member manifesting symptoms of HIV disease from the rest of the family may be appropriate, but the welfare of the infected individual usually is linked intimately to the entire family. Such decisions will be made by physicians and child welfare agencies.

It is widely acknowledged that the number of children with symptoms of HIV disease is growing at an alarming rate. The official count of pediatric AIDS cases significantly understates the true scope of the problem. This situation exists because the criteria for an AIDS diagnosis among children under 13 years differs in important ways from the inclusion criteria for an AIDS diagnosis among adolescents and adults.[20] For example, in the Houston Standard Metropolitan Statistical Area (SMSA) as of October, 1989, less than 30 children under 13 years were reported officially with an AIDS diagnosis, yet pediatricians report they are caring for over 130 infants and children with illnesses related to presumed or confirmed HIV-related diagnoses.[21] It is reasonable to assume that the situation in Houston parallels those in other urban areas in which HIV infections in women and their children constitute a major public health crisis.

Because the incidence of HIV disease in women and children is disproportionately high among blacks and Hispanics, Care Team members from predominantly white congregations may expect to encounter some difficulties in relating to these families because of racial and other possible social, educational, religious, or cultural differences. As a rule of thumb, open, honest expressions of one's lack of familiarity with a client's culture can help to put each person at ease. This acknowledgement can create a mutually instructive atmosphere in which effective, sensitive communication can occur.

In addition to barriers to ministry associated with these factors, Care Teams working with families typically encounter the family's intense concern for privacy and secrecy. This concern is similar to that generally found among adults with HIV disease, but differs to the extent that families are concerned about the impact of disclosure on an ill child or upon other children who are not diagnosed with HIV disease. Assurances of confidentiality are always appropriate, particularly when ministering to families. Considerations of confidentiality also underscore the importance of determining which children in the home have been informed of the nature of a sibling's illness. Team members should inquire of parents what information children may be given, if they ask about the illness of a brother or sister. Parents' wishes should be respected, because this matter is their prerogative. Violation of their wishes not only would contravene the very purpose of the Care Team's ministry and perhaps lead to termination of the caring relationship, but disclosure of sensitive information may cause real harm to the family.

Team members may encounter families whose structures, values, and coping skills are diverse as a result of their unique family background. It should be remembered that the ministries of Care Teams to people touched by AIDS are to be non-judgmental and supportive of pre-existing caring relationships in the family. Families facing AIDS may be suspicious of "authority figures" or "outsiders" who offer to help them during a period of adversity. Some people consider HIV infection an indication of moral failure and parental incompetency. Although these judgments ought not be shared by team members, clients may have this perception. Parents may worry that "the authorities" may seek to remove their children because of reports that the children are being neglected because a parent has AIDS, or a belief that "good parents" would not conceive children if the possibility of HIV infection exists. These fears may be overcome as a Care Team supports a family and respects the integrity of the family unit and the authority of the parents. Team members may find it difficult to maintain a supportive, respectful, and non-judgmental posture, since people tend to be very protective of children. Self-discipline may be required in order to maintain the relationship with the family as a condition for providing care to the children.

If a team member becomes concerned about the welfare of children or parents, the team leader and the service coordinator should be informed. They can address their concerns to the family in a supportive and loving manner, with an offer to assist them in securing additional resources to meet their needs. A conversation with the child's physician may help to relieve a team member's anxieties about a child's welfare. The physician may be able to determine whether the child's condition is due to disease progression or the incapacity of the parents.

Working with families may require a special measure of sensitivity and judgment on the part of team members. Care for a family will involve responding to the concerns and needs of parents and of all children in the home. Parents may share with team members their anticipation of the child's death and grieve that they will not see their child grow to adulthood. Members may have the opportunity to assist parents in working through their grief, which may be accompanied by expressions of guilt because they were the source of infection. They may also be grieving over the prospect that surviving children may be orphaned. Parents may speak of their questions about how to inform a child of his or her AIDS diagnosis or that of a parent, and how to inform uninfected children about a sibling's or parent's diagnosis. They may explore with team members how to provide for their children and plan alternate care.

One of the more emotionally volatile aspects of working with families with AIDS is the discovery that a mother who has already given birth to one HIV-seropositive child is pregnant and planning to bring the pregnancy to term. There is a tendency to judge this as irresponsible behavior, and, perhaps, a moral wrong imposed upon the prospective child. It is important for team members not to express these judgments to a mother to whom they are ministering. There may be many reasons why a woman intends to continue the pregnancy to term. Among those frequently cited is a desire for a child who may, in fact, not be infected. Recent data suggest that the possibility of a newborn being infected is 30 to 50 percent. For women who have lived with much adversity, a 50 to 70 percent chance that this pregnancy will result in a healthy baby who will be a memorial to her may appear quite attractive. Other women may continue pregnancies because of religious beliefs regarding abortion, pressure from family members, fear of abandonment by husbands or partners, or fear of physical abuse. Women may continue pregnancies, even at the risk of transmission to children, as an expression of love for partners. Team members who do not share these reasons or the values inherent in them may be disposed to moralize and make judgments about the people to whom they are ministering. Understanding and restraint may be necessary in these situations because of the tendency of observers to consider children as vulnerable people whom all adults are obliged to protect against harm.

Sympathy for children with HIV disease can be a powerful motivation to care for them and their families. Certain clinical features of infants with HIV disease may heighten sympathy and the tendency to be protective. For example, they may be characterized by their physicians as developmentally delayed or failing to thrive, and may suffer from nutritional deficits, chronic bacterial infections, and experience excessive diarrhea. Their appearance may be distorted by abdominal swelling. These clinical features may present a compelling image to volunteers that elicits an emotional, protective response. Members should note, however, that many infants with HIV disease appear quite normal. They may have all the energy and interests of children their age. Their care and support will be governed by their specific health status and social circumstances.

Team members should be careful not to neglect other children in the home. There is a tendency to focus attention on the child(ren) with HIV disease. Well children have their own needs for attention and love, and members should be alert to indications of anger or jealousy from siblings due to the attention being given to a brother or sister with AIDS. *The importance of always seeing the family unit as the client cannot be overemphasized.* This means in addition that care should be taken to see that well adults are not overlooked. Care-givers may be prone to focus their attention on family members who are ill, with the result that other adults may feel taken for granted. The quality time that team members give to well family members may be reflected in a renewed commitment to and support of those who are ill by well family members. Teams members may also act as sitters so that parents are able to have time away from their family. Sensitivity, open communication, and skill are key characteristics of a comprehensive supportive ministry to families with AIDS.

The physical care of infants and young children with HIV disease does not differ greatly from that provided to children with other illnesses. Team members should follow infection control regimens, for example, washing hands before and after nursing procedures. Children with HIV disease appear to have a heightened susceptibility to bacterial infections. Many infants and young children will have prescribed stimulation therapies, which their primary care providers have been taught to employ. These exercises, which are specially designed for each patient, can also be taught by parents to team members, who can thus relieve parents of these functions. They can be fun activities that also have a therapeutic value.

We recommend that program coordinators and team leaders seek the assistance of a pediatric nurse to design and implement a training program for Care Teams assigned to the care of pediatric AIDS patients. Many adults and parents frequently learn much from pediatric nurses about the proper way to feed, bathe, nurse, and medicate sick infants and young children. (Team members ought not to be overconfident regarding their knowledge of how to care for infants; on the other hand, team members need not be overawed by this responsibility).

There are several guidelines that Care Team members should follow when serving families with HIV disease:

1. It should always be remembered that children with HIV disease are children first, with all the characteristics of "normal" children, except for the limitations imposed by their disease. They may be "well kids" for longer periods than they are "sick kids." Pediatricians recommend that they remain in their home environment as long as possible and that they are treated as much as possible as "normal" children. This mainstreaming approach supports the child and respects the parent-child bond and the role and authority of parents.

2. Team members should be just as clear and direct concerning the limits of their support and care of the family as they would be with other AIDS clients/patients. Setting appropriate limits safeguards against overidentifying with the families served, and against efforts that may be made by families to exploit the services of team members. The team's involvement with the family can thus be directed toward empowering the family to retain control in a situation fraught with problems.

3. Long-term relationships with families under the team's care may include being present as, one by one, HIV-infected family members die. This intense and extended involvement increases the importance of the ministry that team members bear toward each other. Careful attention to one another's needs, especially those related to grief, will be repaid in strengthened bonds between members, and more effective ministry to those whom we serve.

The Shape of Ministry to People Living With AIDS

As we stand at the end of the first AIDS decade and look down the road into the 1990s, details about the AIDS pandemic are becoming clearer:

1. The remarkable surge in research into the structure and function of the virus has opened new vistas of understanding in the field of virology. But equally clear is the world-wide scope of

the danger, which threatens developed and developing countries with equal ferocity.

2. Research into the psychosocial impact of AIDS upon individuals and their communities is enabling social scientists to comprehend the needs of people who are HIV positive or who are living with AIDS, and to fashion responsible, caring responses to them.

3. The religious community is emerging as a source of support for people living with AIDS. Our start may have been belated, but community leadership from responsible religious spokespeople at each level of community life may be determinative in shaping public opinion and attitudes as we enter the 1990s.

The congregational Care Team concept is presented as one avenue by which religious communities can generate pastoral response, effective education, and prophetic leadership in the face of the AIDS crisis. To recognize a crisis one faces is to be confronted by opportunities. Seldom in our lifetimes have the people of God faced such a crisis and such opportunities for ministry. In this context we now explore the shape that ministry may take, and its meaning for people who will be drawn into this area of service.

NOTES

1. Centers for Disease Control, *HIV/AIDS Surveillance Report* (November, 1989).
2. Richard M. Selik, K. G. Castro, and M. Pappaioanou, "Racial/Ethnic Differences in the Risk of AIDS in the United States," *The American Journal of Public Health* 78 (December 1988), 1539-1545; see also James W. Curran, et al., "Epidemiology of HIV Infection and AIDS in the United States," *Science* 239 (February 5, 1988), 610-616.
3. Centers for Disease Control, *HIV/AIDS Surveillance Report* (November, 1989), p. 10.
4. Ibid., p. 9.
5. See Ronald H. Sunderland and Earl E. Shelp, *AIDS: A Manual for Pastoral Care* (Philadelphia: The Westminster Press, 1987), ch. 2; also Earl E. Shelp and Ronald H. Sunderland, *AIDS and the Church* (Philadelphia: The Westminster Press, 1987); chs. 1, 2.
6. Personal communications from health care providers in two Midwest cities, one being a major metropolitan area with a population over one million, and the second a small rural community under twenty-five thousand people.
7. Centers for Disease Control, *AIDS/HIV Surveillance Report* (January, 1990), p. 10.
8. Patrick J. Mason, Roberta A. Olson, and Kathy L. Parish, "AIDS, Hemophilia, and

Prevention Efforts Within a Comprehensive Care Program," *American Psychologist* 43 (November 1988), 971-976.

9. "Medical Aspects of Hemophilia and AIDS," *Focus: A Guide to AIDS Research* (San Francisco: The AIDS Health Project, University of California, 1988), p. 1.

10. "Counseling Issues for People with Hemophilia and HIV Infection," *Focus: A Guide to AIDS Research* (San Francisco: The AIDS Health Project, University of California, 1988), p. 3.

11. Mason, "AIDS, Hemophilia, and Prevention Efforts Within a Comprehensive Care Program," p. 972.

12. Ibid., p. 973.

13. Ibid., p. 974.

14. David Agle, Henry Gluck, and Glenn F. Pierece, "The Risk of AIDS: Psychological Impact on the Hemophilic Population," *General Hospital Psychiatry* 9 (1987); 11-17.

15. Noah D. Cohen et al., "Transmission of Retroviruses by Transfusion of Screened Blood in Patients Undergoing Cardiac Surgery," *The New England Journal of Medicine* 320 (May 4, 1989), 1172-1176.

16. Centers for Disease Control, "Update: AIDS Associated with Intravenous-Drug Use—United States," *Morbidity and Mortality Weekly Report* 38 (March 17, 1989), 165-170.

17. Ibid.

18. For a more detailed discussion of these concerns, see Barbara G. Faltz and Joanna Rinaldi, *AIDS and Substance Abuse: A Training Manual for Health Care Professionals* (San Francisco: The AIDS Health Project, University of California, 1988). This is an indispensable resource for AIDS care-givers. Copies may be ordered ($25.00 plus $2.50 freight) from UCSF AIDS Health Project, Box 0884, San Francisco, CA 94943-0884.

19. Selected References:
Stephane Blanche, et al., "A Prospective Study of Infants Born to Women Seropositive for Human Immunodeficiency Virus Type 1," *New England Journal of Medicine* 320 (June 22, 1989), 1643-1648; Samuel L. Katz and Catherine M. Wilfert, "Human Immunodeficiency Virus Infection of Newborns," *New England Journal of Medicine* 320 (June 22, 1989), 1687-1689; Peter A. Selwyn, et al., "Knowledge of HIV Antibody Status and Decisions to Continue or Terminate Pregnancy Among Intravenous Drug Users," *Journal of the American Medical Association* 261 (June 23/30, 1989), 3567-3571; Judy Macks, "Women and AIDS: Countertransference Issues," *Social Casework* (June 1988), pp. 340-47; George Lewart, "Children and AIDS," *Social Casework* (June 1988), pp. 348-54; Leon G. Epstein, Leroy R. Sharer, and Jaap Goudsmit, "Neurological and Neuropathological Features of Human Immunodeficiency Virus Infection in Children," *Annals of Neurology* 23 (supplement, 1988), 247-68; Stephen D. Barbour, "Acquired Immunodeficiency Syndrome of Childhood," *Pediatric Clinics of North America* 34 (February, 1987), 247-68; Dorothy Ward-Wimmer, "Nursing Care of Children with HIV Infection," *Nursing Clinics of North America* 23 (December 1988), 719-29; Brent G. H. Waters, "The Psychosocial Consequences of Childhood Infection with Human Immunodeficiency Virus," *Medical Journal of Australia* 149 (August 15, 1988), 198-202; Mary Boland, "Practical Aspects of Caring for Children with AIDS," *AIDS in Children, Adolescents and Heterosexual Adults*, Raymond F. Schinazi and Andre J. Nahmias, eds. (New York: Elsevier Science Publishing Co., 1988), pp. 282-85; Nancy Karthas and Anne Dowell, "The Children's AIDS Program: Nursing Challenges," *AIDS in Children, Adolescents and Heterosexual Adults*, Raymond Schinazi and Andre Nahmias, eds. (New York: Elsevier Science Publishing Co., 1988), pp. 288-89.

20. See Institute of Medicine, National Academy of Sciences, *Confronting AIDS: Update 1988* (Washington: National Academy Press, 1988), pp. 208 ff.

21. Personal communication.

CHAPTER SIX

Social, Emotional, and Spiritual Support

People living with HIV disease may be abandoned by family members and ostracized by former acquaintances. HIV disease is a stigmatized condition, and those who experience its impact are often lonely, perhaps because their previous support system is wearing out, or because they have become isolated from it. People who learn they are HIV antibody positive often retreat into a fear-filled and threatened world, withdrawing from people to whom they have been close. The onset of symptoms may be accompanied by an even deeper sense or foreboding, as the person encounters infections, tumors, or other complications resulting from the growing frequency of incapacitating illnesses and hospitalizations.

People with HIV disease may seek increased emotional intimacy and physical contact. These needs are intensified by ignorance of HIV disease and rejection by communities in general or by particular individuals or groups to which the person had looked unavailingly for support.

The acceptance and sensitivity offered by Care Team members are fundamental to building trusting relationships in which care may be offered and accepted without threatening the privacy and autonomy of clients, the integrity of team members or the validity and value of team-client relationships. The resulting strengthened relationships invite a growing level of trust and affirm that people living with AIDS are persons of worth.

Social Support

Support may include:

a. companionship; for example, visiting clients in their homes;
b. inviting clients to visit the member's home/family and Care Team functions;
c. social outings; for example, theater, museum, park, sporting events;
d. accompanying the client to shop for food or other needs.

Any activity that contributes to the health and well-being of clients affirms them as persons and strengthens their sense of autonomy. This perception of self-control will benefit them. The support services outlined above may be complemented by other acts of thoughtfulness that reinforce the message which team members provide through their ministry out of love and compassion. These may include:

a. daily household tasks such as watering plants, exercising a pet and caring for the pet when the patient is in the hospital;
b. a visit on a holiday, decorating the home, or bringing flowers;
c. celebrating birthdays;
d. helping with mail and correspondence, including payment of bills;
e. encouraging and assisting the patient to ambulate, including walks outside the home, if feasible.

These activities are relationship-building, the type of companionship and care one friend offers another.

Emotional Support

Social activities can be a first step toward extending emotional support to clients. Because HIV disease tends to be accompanied by progressive debility and dependence, its psychological consequences may be as devastating as the disease itself. Diagnosis with HIV disease tends to set in motion a transition from a healthy, normal life-style to being weakened and infection-prone. The fact that HIV may be dormant for a lengthy period may afford some ease of mind, but the fear of developing symptoms of catastrophic disease is rarely absent. Diminished self-esteem, depression, and suicidal thoughts are not uncommon. Patients or family members may be angry, and the normal stresses that exist in family constellations may be exacerbated. The social support outlined above may be supplemented by observing the following:

a. Encourage clients to set their own agendas, thereby reinforcing their autonomy.

b. Develop a listening style, inviting clients to share their stories to the extent they desire.

c. Remember that team members cannot change the realities clients face or assume responsibility to resolve their problems. One important contribution may be to suggest and explore options from which clients or care-providers may choose in making decisions. Members should not feel guilty that they cannot change the reality facing people living with AIDS.

d. Team members will affirm the personhood and dignity of clients by assisting them to sort through options, suggesting possible actions open to them, and offering practical aid (transportation to a clinic or relevant city, county, or Social Security office).

Imagination and common sense will suggest other forms of support. Such support may be one of the most important gifts Care Team members can offer.

The Ministry of Clients to Team Members

Team-client relationships cannot be reduced merely to the presumption that clients' needs are the occasion for ministry offered by team members. In addition to the ministry team members offer clients, people living with HIV disease may offer an important ministry to team members. In the intense relationships that develop between clients and team members, care-providers may be enriched by gifts clients bring to the relationships, if each is open to the other. For example, the courage of clients in the face of HIV disease, as well as their own religious pilgrimages, may contribute to care-givers' lives by opening up new possibilities for self-exploration and growth, both emotionally and spiritually. (See pp. 58–60) Team members should remain sensitive and open to other aspects of team-client relationships through which clients may minister to them; ministry is always a two-way street.

Spiritual Support

People living with HIV disease often seek renewal of previous religious ties, or may initiate a relationship with a faith group for the first time. The decision may be made to move from a former denomination to another denomination that is perceived to meet the person's needs more completely.[1] While not every person to whom team members minister will have or express spiritual needs, there will often be opportunities to share religious experiences and values. The initiative to raise these issues always remains with the clients, in order to avoid any appearance that care-givers are taking advantage of the vulnerable situation in which clients find themselves. Every effort should be made to maintain and enhance the self-esteem and dignity of people living with HIV disease, and the exercise of care in these matters is paramount.

These discussions may begin with a comment from the client, for example:

Client: Why are you here?
Member: I'm here because I care about you, and I want to help, if I am able. That is what my faith teaches is important.

> **Client:**   What does faith have to do with this?
> **Member:** If my faith isn't expressed in some service to others, it seems to me that it is incomplete.

The offering of this level of care is itself a pastoral ministry. It witnesses to the team member's own religious experience and values, and may lead to discussion of the member's motives. The following suggestions may facilitate this process:

a. Sharing social outings and events with clients, for some teams, has included inviting clients to participate in team gatherings. This has assisted in the development of strong bonds between clients and team members, leading some clients to express the wish to attend other congregational activities, including worship. This latter initiative should remain with the client, not with the team member.

b. Discussion of spiritual issues may lead to a request for assistance in reestablishing contacts with a client's own faith group, for example, making provision for a visit by a clergy person from a client's faith group.

c. Consistency and loyalty are paramount attributes in any relationship, but are more than usually important in relationships with people living with HIV disease. Care that is given to keeping schedules, commitment to each client, and affirming the client as a person of worth speak to the integrity of the spiritual witness offered by team members.

The Pastoral Identity of Team Members

Ministry to people living with HIV disease is offered in a climate shaped in part by fears and negative moral attitudes in the general public, poor medical prognoses, and harsh social judgments associated with AIDS. It is difficult for Care Team members to remain untouched by such influences. Such factors may cause team members to examine their own faith, and to be ready to address their own emotional and religious questions and crises.[2]

Pastoral ministry is shaped by two factors: the "pastoral identity" of the minister (lay or ordained) and the pastoral or spiritual needs of the person to whom care is offered. Pastoral identity is a term usually applied to clergy. It signifies the minister's awareness of gifts or aptitudes which equip that person to offer pastoral ministry. But the minister's self-awareness is evaluated by that of the community—in this case, the congregation. Members who feel drawn to ministry to people living with HIV disease must satisfy the congregation that they are suited for this ministry. This may be determined by the pastor, priest, or rabbi, or by a designated committee, a process which constitutes an appropriate screening of lay participants.

Pastoral ministry encompasses a wide range of pastoral services, including visitation and companionship in informal settings, as outlined under "Social Support" above, and extending to spiritual conversation and worship. It is the visitors' sense that they offer these ministries in response to their pastoral call that imbues these activities with "pastoral" meaning. Such ministry, however, is a gift, offered in response to the needs of clients, which loses its pastoral identity if imposed on the clients. The person receiving ministry must be free to decline offered help. Hence, the Care Team program has integrity only when it is non-abusive, non-exploitive, and non-judgmental. Thus, for example, proselytism is excluded from ministry.

The ministry of reconciliation is closely identified with spiritual nurture, and may take the form of renewed religious life, as indicated above, or renewal of relationships with families and friends. Team members have recounted incidents in which their presence in a client's home during visits of family members has assisted in renewing ties between parents or siblings and their client. They have noted the surprise of family members at the presence of team members, and their curiosity at the scope and commitment of the Care Team's activities, opening the door to discussion of their ministry.

Involvement of lay people in the provision of pastoral ministry not only provides care for people in need of acceptance, reassurance, and love, which is the reason for the very existence of the Care Team program, but also offers an opportunity in the care-givers' own lives at which their own spiritual formation is extended and deepened. Each person both gives and receives, and each is blessed. This may be the case especially when team members are ministering to a patient whose death is imminent. This is one of the most poignant aspects of ministry, and one for which team members should prepare, both within the team membership, and, where appropriate, with the dying patient.

Team members whose experience extends for up to three years have found that funeral planning may assume growing importance for patients as they weaken and confront the reality of death.[3] Some patients have invited team members to assist in writing the funeral service, and teams frequently participate in the subsequent rites. Members of congregations in Houston have traveled to cities such as El Paso and Corpus Christi, and as far away as Wisconsin, to share with families in the funerals of former patients.

Ministry When the Patient Dies

1. Some patients die in a hospital, nursing home, or hospice. If the patient has been moved to an acute or extended care facility, it is assumed that Care Team members will maintain ministry though visitation. Following the patient's death, team members have their own grief work to do (see Chapter 4), as well as attending to the needs of family or friends of the patient when that is appropriate.

2. Some patients will choose to die at home. In this event, the Care Team should function in a supporting role, providing emotional support to the household, perhaps bringing meals and running errands. It is often feasible (and the patient may request this continuing ministry) for the team members to continue physical care, e.g., bathing and oral hygiene. Remember that the Basic Nursing Skills section of this document is written with this in mind.

   a. The Care Team may seek special training from the service coordinator and the nursing consultants with whom they work to provide these hospice-like care activities. Alternately, a local hospice may provide this element of training to members, teaching members how to keep the dying person comfortable.

b. Team members may assist clients by enabling them to control their dying as much as they have wanted to control their lives.

c. Teams should balance the support of the dying patient, the family members, and the friends with whom the patient wishes to retain contact, calling upon the service coordinator for assistance and guidance, as needed.

d. Team members should keep in mind that they are to work within the limits of what the patient and family desire, on the one hand, and what team members are able to provide, on the other. They should consult with the team leader when tension or conflict arises, remembering that anger may accompany grief.

e. Team members remain guests in the homes of those to whom they minister. Thus, they may be requested to leave. When team members have given of themselves, they should be ready to let the family or lover remain with the dying patient in privacy. The patient may need to reduce the number of people in the intimate circle of family and friends, and the most loving act on the part of team members may be to "die to self."

f. Nevertheless, our experience suggests that, as death becomes imminent, the patient and family depend on the Care Team even more. It is important, therefore, to anticipate how team members will respond to the events surrounding a patient's death.

g. A further word of support to team members: The team is a part of a total care function which in many instances may have been shared with members of the patient's family and other friends. It is not the team members' responsibility to respond to *every* need or demand.

3. Team members may help by bringing the following issues to the attention of the patient or the primary care-providers responsible for decisions related to the death of the patient:

    a. It is appropriate to anticipate such decisions as selection of a funeral director. The patient may already have made this decision.

    b. The patient or primary care-provider(s) should have available a list of names and phone numbers of people to be contacted when the patient dies, including:
- The home nursing service, if applicable, or the patient's physician;
- Family members or close friends whom the patient wishes to be kept informed.

    c. It is in the patient's interests for the Care Team to be familiar with the regimen of patient care that has been agreed upon by the patient and the primary care-providers. Information may include what supportive medical steps have been approved by the patient and prescribed by the physician, and what comfort measures have been approved, so that there is no misunderstanding of the actions to be taken, for example, if the patient goes into pulmonary or cardiac arrest, and dies.

4. When death occurs, team members who are present should assist the person(s) responsible for decisions to:

    a. Notify the home nursing service, which should call the physician or mortician.

    b. Call either the patient's physician or the mortician, one of whom will report the death to the coroner, if a home nursing service has not been attending the patient.

5. After the client dies:

    a. If present when the coroner releases the body, team members may offer one of their most caring and sensitive ministries by preparing the body to be viewed by loved ones, leaving the body as esthetically pleasing as possible so that they may see the body in the most gracious way (the hair can be combed, medications removed, IV poles removed, the face wiped clean, and so forth). This may be particularly appreciated if the body will not be viewed again.

b. Team members may remain to support the survivors. If possible, they may arrange to provide continuing care. For example, the team may have access to families in the congregation who can provide meals and other support.

c. In general, team members should be careful not to take charge and rush events and people. Members should inform survivors of their availability to remain with the family or lover, or, if they must leave, the possibility, in consultation with the team leader, of calling upon other team members.

6. Care Team members cannot maintain intense, pastoral relationships with every family group of survivors. Though there may be some situations in which close contact continues, in general, closure is appropriate and advisable.

a. Some family members, after an appropriate period, may ask to share in the team's ministry. Team leaders should respond as they would to any inquiry concerning participation in the team's work.

b. If family members need continuing grief support, there may be a grief support ministry sponsored by the congregation into which they may be integrated, or the congregation may be challenged to develop such a ministry as one of its functions.

c. Referring survivors to a separate support system allows the team members to focus on their specialized ministry.

d. Team members should be in touch with their own grief, seek support from group members as needed, and be alert to the grief of other members who were close to the dying patient.

Support of Family and Friends

Much of the content of this book refers to care of the person living with AIDS but applies equally to ministry to family members and friends. For example, provision of social, emotional, and spiritual support of the types indicated is just as important for the circle of family and friends as for the client. This is particularly applicable to grief ministry.

When a family is confronted with a serious illness or disability, its members usually are faced with a radical disruption of relationships, roles, and the stability and sense of security to which the family was accustomed prior to the health crisis. The disruption is experienced by everyone: parents, siblings, adult children (whether in the home or not), relatives, and friends. In the case of AIDS, this situation may be exacerbated even more by the needs of family members to maintain secrecy not only from friends but from other family members. This effort may be extremely taxing on the inner circle of the family, because it entails both the effort to restrict information and the fear that, despite the best efforts, others may learn the family member's status.

The emotional and physical burden of coping with these threats may be overwhelming. New roles adopted to cope with the crisis of AIDS may produce new stresses between family members, or exacerbate existing, unresolved intra-family stresses. For example, when John's parents urged him to return from Los Angeles so that they could care for him in their home, both participated in that decision. However, six months later, John's father moved to the guest bedroom as John's medical crisis deepened and he required constant care. John's father could not tolerate caring for John in the home and he began to resent the extent to which John's care preoccupied his wife. Within six months, John's parents had separated. While this account may be unusual in its severity, it illustrates the extent of the impact that the care of a chronically ill patient may have upon family relationships.

Even in those instances in which a family draws together to

meet the crisis, using all its resources to support the person with AIDS, disruption may still be catastrophic. When families face intense health threats, the needs of members may diverge. A formerly independent person may become dependent upon the care and support of others, and care-providers may adopt parental attitudes toward the disabled member. Families ill-prepared for crises may have to deal with the patient's growing physical and emotional dependence, often complicated by worsening AIDS dementia.

Increasingly people with AIDS are experiencing neurological and mental conditions similar to those associated with Alzheimer's disease. For example, AIDS dementia may begin to appear in the forms of short term memory loss, transient confusion, difficulty with coordination, and difficulty with motor skills. The symptoms may deteriorate over time, improve, or stabilize. In addition to the implications of these symptoms for providing supportive care, people with AIDS frequently are aware of these mental and neurological losses. Their perception that they might lose these faculties and capabilities may evoke anger and frustration, which might be displaced to care providers. At times, psychiatric conditions are seen concurrently with these types of neurological losses. Accordingly, a frightening situation to patients and care-givers can become even more distressing. Care providers may be required to exercise even greater patience and firmness in relating to clients. These neurologic and psychiatric developments often result in the client's increased dependence on others and a need for increased supervision. As a consequence, care-givers may experience more fatigue and stress related to the heightened attention that the client requires. Care-givers may also become more concerned about their capacity to maintain an increasing level of care and a near total devotion to the client. In short, these developments may result in AIDS "consuming" everyone within reach. Care Team members should be sensitive to the impact on the client and his or her family, as well as on fellow team members.

The stress of adapting to the changed situation in the family may evoke feelings of grief, which may be expressed in numerous forms. In particular, family members may resort to denial or experience anger and deepening sadness. These responses are often manifested in intense intra-personal conflicts, of which the following are characteristic.

Affection versus resentment: Care-providers responsible for intensifying patient support may care out of affection for their loved one, yet still feel resentful because of the demands now being made upon them. It is often difficult to manage the ambivalence inherent in this situation, and corresponding feelings of guilt may be experienced. Care Team members should be alert to the needs of family members and lovers, and both listen for and respond to such feelings, and provide reassurance that these feelings are "normal."

Companionship versus isolation: Growing physical and emotional needs on the part of a patient, accompanied by diverging needs of patient and care-provider, may lead to growing emotional distance between the two. Further, the necessity to make extensive time commitments to patient care may result in isolation of the care-provider from customary sources of support. This is intensified if attempts are made to keep HIV infection a close family secret.

Loneliness may also be heightened if the presence in the home of a person with AIDS causes care-providers to forgo significant relationships. Family members may become increasingly lonely if unable to maintain activities, especially those functions in which they participated previously.

Care Team members' support of family members may be decisive in enabling them to recognize their dilemma and to strengthen the support system that is in place. The presence of Care Team members offers care-providers opportunities to enhance social and other relationships, which will be important when family members or lovers must adapt to their new situations following the death of the patient.

Patience versus frustration: Regardless of the warmth and strength of the relationship between patient and care-provider, family members or lovers may become discouraged when the patient shows little progress toward the desired health, or when one more crisis and hospitalization serves as a painful reminder that the disease is taking its toll. The discouragement is characterized by additional anguish if AIDS dementia complicates an already frustrating situation. Again, the reassurance by Care Team members that the care-provider's feelings are "normal" and understandable may do much to relieve fear and anxiety.

Independence versus dependence: There is a fine line separating care that encourages independence and care that manipulates the patient into a dependent relationship. Care Team members should be alert to this risk both in themselves and in family members. If noted, it should be pointed out as a behavior that may not best serve the interests or needs of the patient.

Hope versus despair: Frequent, rapid changes in medical status is one of the characteristics of the course of HIV progressive disease. A sudden crisis is likely to plunge the care-provider into despair. Yet a short time later, the patient may show a remarkable improvement in status, and hope quickly replaces fear. This emotional "roller-coaster" is likely to be exhausting for both care-provider and patient, and may be accompanied by some or all of the emotions identified in this section: impatience, guilt, denial, frustration, and so forth. Once more, team members' openness to families may play a significant part in enabling them to recognize and understand these events as they occur, and to process them so that they do not immobilize care-providers.

Letting go versus holding on: As medical crises become more frequent and more intense, anticipation of separation through death is inevitable. The primary care-providers may intensify efforts to cope through denial, resulting in exhaustion, impatience, frustration, and hope that is buoyed only by strenuous effort, or they must begin the painful process of "letting go." They may vacillate between guilt evoked by a wish that their ordeal would end and the anticipated relief of being spared the day-to-day responsibilities of providing care, on one hand, and their inability to let go of their dying family member, on the other. Team members may assist family members in breaking this cycle of grief by helping them to recognize and acknowledge their ambivalence, thus affirming the validity of their feelings, and enabling them to begin the painful work of grieving. In turn, family members may be empowered to give their dying member "permission" to die. Team members may also be able to address care-providers' needs by initiating discussion of how they are planning to deal with the patient's death and the subsequent changes in their lifestyles.

Response to *anticipatory* grief is similar to caring for people in grief. When undertaken sensitively, the team's grief ministry may help care-providers to be self-conscious about grieving without the more negative effects of ambivalence.

Other Aspects of Ministry with Families

The following suggests some appropriate ministry responses to the needs of clients' parents or other family members:

1. If they arrive in the city from out of town, services may include meeting them at the airport or being at the client's home when they arrive.
2. Some parents may learn in the same conversation that their son is gay or that their son or daughter is an IV drug user and is HIV antibody positive or has AIDS. Team members' support may make the difference in the way parents hear and understand this information. For example, if one parent is excessively distressed, it may help to talk to this parent in another room. Remember that one of the initial responses may be grief, which is often expressed as anger.
3. When family members are involved as care-providers, it is just as important to be clear about team members' roles and functions with them. It is wise to be specific with respect to clarifying any limits upon which the team and the client have agreed. The division of services between family members (or lover or friend) should be specifically

delineated. The client should be consulted and the client's reasonable wishes respected to the extent possible.

4. Team members should always check with clients to learn which family members are aware of the diagnosis, what others know, or what clients wish others to know. Clients have the right to limit communication to those people who have a "need to know." Team members must honor these wishes and be careful to avoid disclosing information not sanctioned by clients.

5. It is important for adults with HIV disease to remember that young children in the family may be uninhibited in discussing the family's medical status outside the home. Siblings may not hesitate to inform neighbors or school friends that a brother, sister, or parent has AIDS. It is appropriate for team members to discuss and clarify these issues with clients.

The motivation to undertake ministries such as these with people living with AIDS and with members of their families is always rooted in our identity as the people of God. Jewish and Christian scriptures alike are replete with images, no, *mitzvoth* (commandments), to visit and care for the sick and disabled. The notion that God's people are to express their devotion to God in part through their care of people who are unable to care for themselves in inseparable from this identity.[4] It is captured, for example, in the New Testament parable of the Judgment: "I was sick, and you visited me" (Matt. 25:36), and implicit in the Jewish scriptures "You shall open wide your hand to your brother, to the needy and to the poor (Deut. 15:11; see also Deut. 14:29*b*; Job 29:12-13; and Ps. 146: 7-9). The tradition is explicit in its affirmation that such care is to be expressed not in mere pietist wishes of good will, but in the most practical ways. We are to manifest the same love and care to the "needy" (Ps. 9:18) that we have received from God.

As one learns to walk with people living with AIDS, one is likely to find that ministry, which begins with social, emotional, and spiritual support for people in reasonable health, moves inexorably into hospice-level support for patients whose bodies are wasted and their strength dissipated. People in end-stage AIDS may require comprehensive care, including assistance to walk, skin care, and bed-baths if they are bed-ridden. Such ministry is demanding, and not every person is suited to this aspect of Care Team activities. It should be expected that teams may be constituted of persons with a variety of gifts, skills, and abilities. The next chapter delineates a basic nursing care program and guides Care Team members through steps to be taken at each level of care.

NOTES

1. See, for example, "Thelma and Ralph," in Earl E. Shelp, Ronald H. Sunderland, and Peter W. A. Mansell, *AIDS: Personal Stories in Pastoral Perspective* (New York: The Pilgrim Press, 1986), pp. 99-105.
2. For a more complete discussion of these concerns, see Earl E. Shelp and Ronald H. Sunderland, *AIDS and the Church* (Philadelphia: The Westminster Press, 1987), ch. 5.
3. See Elizabeth Goss, "Living and Dying with AIDS," *The Journal of Pastoral Care* 43 (Winter 1989), pp. 297-308.
4. See, for example, Earl E. Shelp and Ronald H. Sunderland, *AIDS and the Church* (Philadelphia: The Westminster Press, 1987), chs. 2, 3; also Samuel E. Karff, "Ministry in Judaism: Reflections on Suffering and Caring," *A Biblical Basis for Ministry*, Earl E. Shelp and Ronald H. Sunderland, eds. (Philadelphia: The Westminster Press, 1981), ch. 2; and Klaus Seybold and Ulrich B. Mueller, *Sickness and Healing* (Nashville: Abingdon Press, 1981).

CHAPTER SEVEN

Activities of Daily Living

People weakened and fatigued by HIV disease may be unable to perform basic functions of daily living. Ministry to people living with AIDS often will take the form of assisting with such routine tasks as house cleaning, meal preparation, and maintaining personal hygiene. Such services must be offered in a manner that does not override the wishes and rights of clients who are probably experiencing loss of control over themselves and their activities. Care-givers will often find their most effective ministry will be encouraging clients to do for themselves what the care-giver could accomplish quicker and more competently, but at the cost of the client's experiences of success in managing his or her own daily chores. Most clients will want to remain independent as long as possible, and current research indicates their health status will benefit from doing so. Team members should encourage clients to set the pace during their visits.

Care for Ambulatory Clients

Relationships between client and team members will be mutually beneficial if simple routines are followed. For example, a weekly schedule may be developed that tabulates clients' needs and the responsibilities of the respective team members. Thus, days may be specified for meal preparation or physician visits. Names of team members assigned to provide transportation may be included. Simple, common-sense guidelines should be followed:

  a. *Meal preparation:* Choices should be made with respect to the client's likes, dislikes, and, of course, dietary and nutritional needs.
  b. *Household tasks:* The client should be consulted regarding other household chores, and personal aspects such as dressing and self-care.
  c. *Shopping:* A client may be unable to go shopping unless accompanied. This is an appropriate activity, meeting practical needs and providing companionship and emotional support.

Team members' activities should be planned to adapt to the changing needs of clients/patients. The most basic criteria for planning are sound judgment, common sense, and sensitivity. It is also important to be open to clients' wishes and needs, including consultation regarding desired or required activities, and how these can be performed. Only activities that affirm the client's dignity, autonomy, and self-esteem should be considered.

Team members will find it helpful to remember that, even with the highest intentions and good will, they will make mistakes, or be misunderstood. It is important to anticipate such events, to be open in acknowledging them, to seek patiently to correct errors, and to achieve common understanding. These attitudes are especially essential when assisting clients/patients with daily living activities.

Basic Nursing Care for Non-Ambulatory Patients

Assisting clients with aspects of personal care—such as bathing, changing bed linen, turning patients in bed, and moving patients to and from bed—is one of the most fundamental and important Care Team activities. It is also one of the most demanding tasks. These tasks are summarized under the phrase *basic nursing care*, which refers to those activities performed for people living with HIV disease who are not fully able to care for themselves.

The term basic nursing care refers to a number of activities that may be undertaken by a trained lay person, including:

bathing
tepid sponging to lower fever
oral hygiene
moving/turning the patient in bed
exercising/mobilization
rubbing/massaging extremities, torso
bowel elimination and continence care
feeding and provision of liquids
changing bed linen when patient is in bed
patient transfer: assisting patient to get out of or into bed
shaving.

Most patients will be familiar with these basic nursing functions from previous experiences in the hospital or the assistance of home health care personnel. Before beginning any procedure, care-givers should:
- discuss the proposed activity with the patient, including his or her general welfare, needs, limitations, and preferences about how a task may be done in comfort;
- inquire how the patient is feeling and what can be accomplished without assistance;
- recognize and affirm the patient's efforts in his or her own behalf.

Giving a bed bath

Patients usually prefer to care for themselves, particularly in respect to bathing; assistance is required only when patients are so physically weak as to be unable to bathe themselves.

Equipment:
  • basin (e.g., hospital issue; approximately 15″ × 12″)
  • kidney basin (hospital issue; suited to brushing teeth and rinsing mouth)
  • water as warm as you can stand; touch with your elbow to test temperature if immersing patient's hands or feet
  • towels, washcloths, and bath blanket or large beach towel.

Procedure

1. Preparation:
   a. Assist the patient to sit up in bed or in a bed-side chair, if able to move (see "Patient Transfer," p. 123).
   b. If patient is immobile, place the large towel or bath blanket over the patient to maintain body temperature, comfort, and privacy.
2. Face:
   a. Wash face first, starting with eyes. Use clear water. Drape the damp wash cloth over the index finger. Beginning at the inner canthus (see Fig. 1), wipe to the outside, using a separate area of the cloth for each eye.
   b. Wash the face, ears, and neck (Fig. 2), using the folded cloth as a mitten (Fig. 2).
3. Remainder of body:
   a. Uncover one part of the body at a time (e.g., left arm). Immerse the folded mitten in water, wring out excess water and lightly soap and wash arm, including axilla (underarm). When bathing the arm, support the arm by tucking the patient's hand under your left arm to hold it in position for washing, using the mitten on your right hand (Fig. 3).
   b. Rinse cloth and carefully wipe off all soap from sponged areas. Dry each area well.
   c. Patients enjoy soaking their hands in the bath water. Test the temperature with your elbow first.
      NOTE: If skin is dry, do not use soap. Patient may use a bath oil in place of soap.
   d. Repeat for other arm, legs, torso. When washing the lower leg lift the leg at the ankle and knee. Support the leg with one arm while sponging with the other hand (Fig. 4, 5).

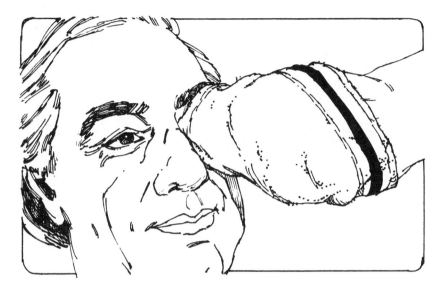

Figure 1

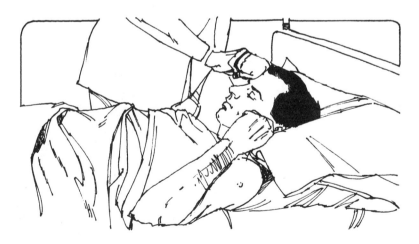

Figure 2

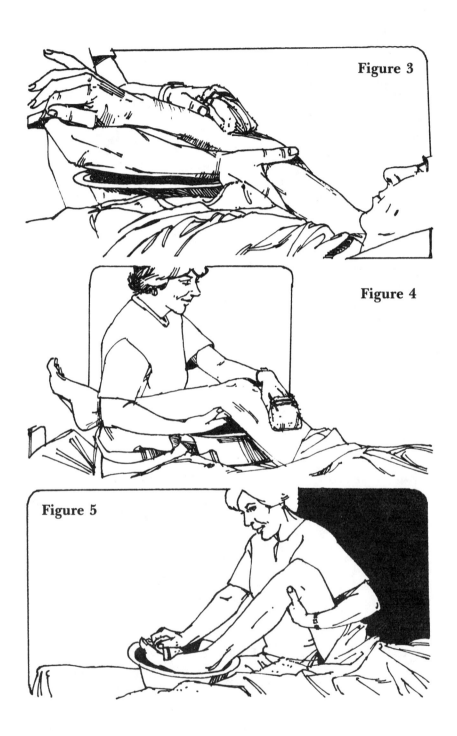

Figure 3

Figure 4

Figure 5

e. Patients enjoy being able to place their feet in a basin of warm water while bed-ridden. Test the water temperature with your elbow. Support the leg at the ankle and knee while placing the foot carefully in the basin (Fig. 5).

NOTE: Check with the patient regularly during bathing procedures to assess body temperature, comfort, and fatigue level. Change the water frequently and avoid dipping soap in water. Always dry sponged areas thoroughly, keeping body covered except for the area being sponged/dried. Patient may be assisted with a tub bath or shower. A shower chair will greatly facilitate a weakened patient to shower with lesser assistance.

f. Anal area (wear gloves for this procedure):

It is important to keep the anal area clean and dry. Roll the patient to side-lying position. Draw upper leg toward the chest to expose anus. (Use two hands to support leg as it is moved.) Wash gently and rinse well. Dry thoroughly, with gentle, dabbing motion. Diarrhea-prone patients may be very sore; if the anal area is inflamed, use an alcohol-free wet-wipe instead of soap and wash cloth.

Tepid Sponging

Employ tepid sponging when the patient's fever is unresponsive to anti-pyretics (i.e., aspirin or Tylenol). The procedure is designed to bring the temperature down slowly. Rapid reduction in temperature causes shivering, which will cause the temperature to rise again. Check with the patient, who will usually know when to worry about temperature control.

Procedure
1. Use a wash cloth formed into a mitten (see above).
2. Keep the bath blanket over body parts not being sponged. Close doors and windows to prevent drafts.
3. Begin with warm water, slightly below body temperature. Equal parts of water and ethyl alcohol may be used.
4. Place wash cloths in water, wring out excess, and place

under each axilla (underarm) and over the groin.

5. Using the mitten, gently sponge an extremity for five minutes. Note the patient's response.

6. Dry the extremity and check patient's temperature and pulse (See steps 12 and 13 below).

7. Continue sponging the other extremities, back, and buttocks for 3–5 minutes each. Reassess temperature and pulse every 15 minutes.

8. Change the water and reapply sponges to the axillae and groin as needed.

9. When the body temperature falls to slightly above normal, discontinue the procedure.

10. Dry the extremities and body parts thoroughly. Cover the patient with a light bath blanket or sheet.

11. Change the bed linen, if needed.

12. Measure the patient's temperature, and record the time the procedure was started and terminated; note vital sign changes and the patient's response for the home-health care service, physician, or other agency. If the temperature is not lowered or does not stay down, a call to the client's physician may be indicated.

13. Pulse rates in adolescents and adults vary from 60 to 100 beats per minute. Check with the patient regarding feelings of discomfort or anxiety associated with variations in rates, and whether to call the physician.

Oral Hygiene

There is aesthetic value as well as comfort in having a clean and healthy mouth, but the important issue is contribution to overall health. To prevent injury or irritation of sore areas, exercise care while cleaning the mouth. Always use a soft tooth brush. Due to their generally debilitated state and the fact that they may be too fatigued to brush their teeth, patients often have fragile gums. Many also have thrush, a yeast infection, or other lesions which make their mouths sore. Patients should also brush their teeth after vomiting, to protect teeth from stomach acids.

Procedure
1. Helper should wear gloves.
2. If the patient is too weak to sit up while brushing teeth, slide the patient in the side-lying position to the side of the bed nearest you, with head turned down toward the mattress. Place a towel under the patient's head and the kidney basin under the patient's chin (Figure 6). (Dentists recommend a tartar-control tooth paste.)
3. In the extreme case in which the patient is unresponsive, hold the mouth open with a padded tongue blade, and substitute a wet toothette (a special sponge toothbrush) for a tooth brush. Clean the mouth using a wet gauze pad wrapped around a tongue blade. (Use a mixture of one-third each Cepacol/Listerine, hydrogen peroxide, and water.)
4. Periodic application of a lip balm is comforting.

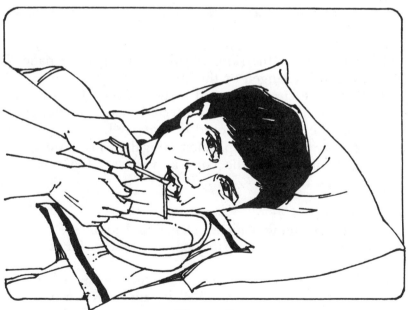

Figure 6

Prevention of Problems Arising from Prolonged Bed Rest

The immobilized patient, unable to meet his/her own hygiene needs, depends on assistance to maintain skin and muscle integrity. A hygiene routine, therefore, should be part of the total care, including the removal of skin bacteria by bathing, regular position changing, encouraging the patient to exercise in bed, joint mobility and massaging. When a patient is unable to turn himself or herself, turning the patient regularly will afford comfort, and help to prevent bed sores (decubitus ulcers).

Decubitus Ulcers

A decubitus ulcer is an inflammation, sore, or ulcer in the skin that covers a bony prominence, for example, heel, elbow, or buttocks (Figure 7). Damage to the skin occurs when circulation is cut off. Pathological changes may occur within an hour from pressure due to the patient's position in bed. The longer the pressure is applied, the greater is the risk of skin breakdown.

Stages of Development
1. Reddening of the skin, which fades when the patient's position is changed or the area is gently massaged.
2. Superficial circulatory and tissue damage. In this stage, redness and swelling of the affected area do not disappear when the patient is moved or massaged.
3. The third stage is deep, penetrating decaying of the tissue, which may affect the bone as well as soft tissues and muscles.

Procedure
1. When handling patient (changing bed linen, bathing, transferring from or to the bed, etc.,) observe for reddened skin areas.
2. Massage gently with lotion or Sween Cream, noting whether redness fades when pressure is relieved.
3. Encourage patient to move around in bed, developing muscle tone through exercise, and relieving pressure points.

4. Report to visiting nurse, home health service, or the patient's family or physician reddened areas that do not disappear when pressure is removed.

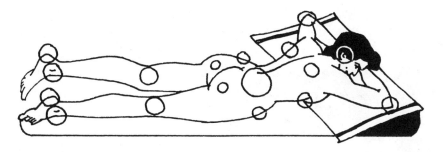

Figure 7

Exercising the Immobilized Patient

Deterioration of muscle can be prevented by assisting patients to exercise in bed. Figures 8-11 illustrate range of motion exercises for arms, and legs and feet.

If patients are not having difficulty breathing and feel strong enough, they may be shown how to exercise their limbs. When patients are unable to undertake exercises unaided, follow these procedures:

Procedure
1. Arm exercising: support the arm at hand and elbow, as in Figs. 8 and 11(a). Gently move arm through field of motion; move each finger tip in turn to touch the tip of the thumb.
2. Leg and foot: support the heel and knee joints as illustrated (Fig. 9). Exercise toes, as in Fig. 10.
3. Flex the hip joint and knee joint with gentle movements, bringing the knee toward the abdomen within comfort ranges.
4. Flex the ankle, while supporting the leg (Fig. 11[b]).

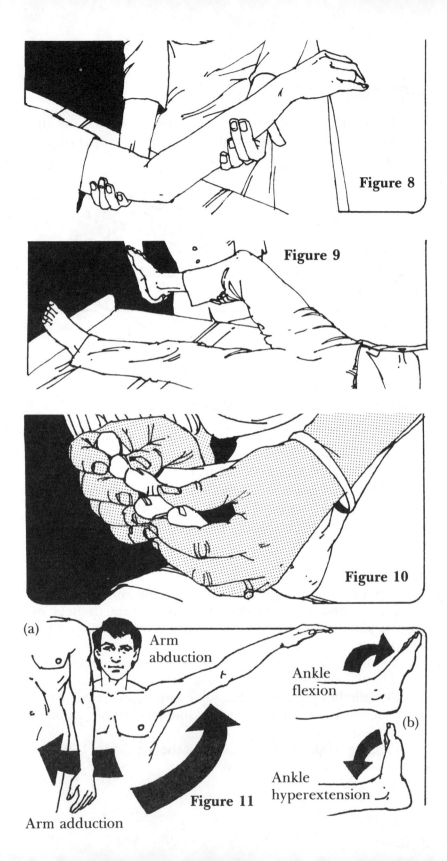

Figure 8

Figure 9

Figure 10

(a)

Arm
abduction

Ankle
flexion

(b)

Arm adduction

Ankle
hyperextension

Figure 11

Rubbing or Massaging the Patient (see illustrations 12-17)

Following the bath or shower, patients enjoy having their hands and feet rubbed. A back rub acts as a general body conditioner, and promotes peripheral circulation. Such treatments can be very relaxing. Because energy is required to keep muscles in tension, for example, when tension is released through rubbing, energy is also released to be redirected to other parts of the body.

Procedure
1. Use a lotion or Sweem Cream. Pour lotion into your hands and warm it before applying to patient by rubbing hands together.
2. Use long, slow strokes along the length of the back, across the deltoid (shoulder) muscles, up the neck and along the shoulders (Figs. 12-14). With the fingers together, keep the hands on the skin at all times, and follow the muscle groups while moving up the neck (Fig. 15). Strokes should be firm but gradually lighter as the rub motion is ending. Encourage the patient to let you know if you should rub harder or softer.
3. Muscle tension may also be relieved with gentle "chopping" motions with the hands (Fig. 16), or "kneading" (Fig. 17).

Moving/Turning the Patient in Bed

Procedure
1. Face the patient and slide the patient toward you. If alone, you can do this in segments: Support the patient's neck and shoulders with both arms, and draw the patient's head and shoulders to the edge of the mattress.
2. Similarly move the patient's legs, then hips (again using both arms to provide maximum comfort; see Fig. 18).

NOTE: This movement can be effected with ease if two people work together.

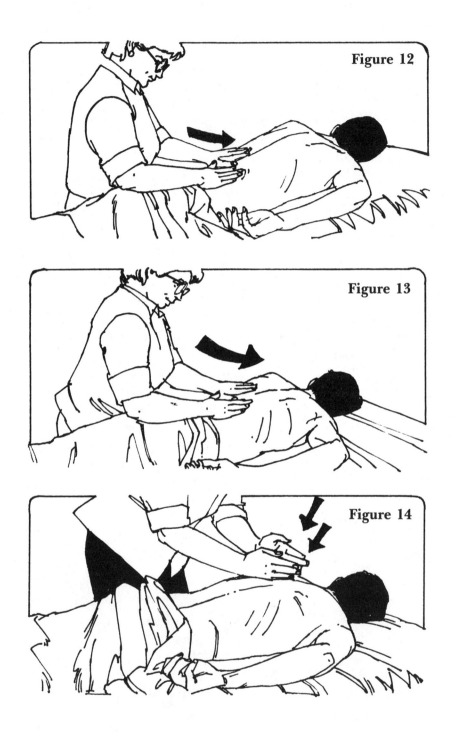

Figure 12

Figure 13

Figure 14

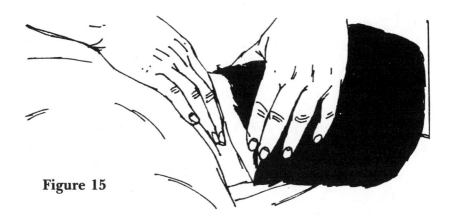

Figure 15

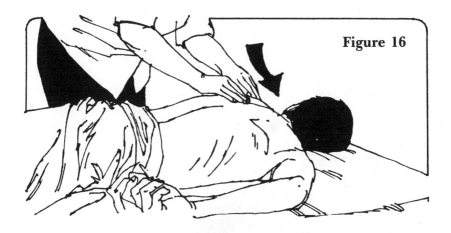

Figure 16

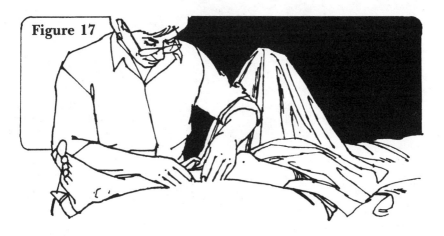

Figure 17

3. Assume a broad stance (feet apart and braced, one in front of the other) facing the patient. Place your upper arm under the patient's shoulders, being careful to support the cervical vertebrae and head. Place the other arm under the patient's thighs.

4. Bending at the waist, roll the patient away from you, toward the center of the bed, rolling the patient onto the side-lying position. The helper can support the upper leg at the knee and ankle.

Alternate method of Turning the Patient

A "turning sheet" is placed in position under the patient, from shoulders to thighs (Fig. 19). The turning sheet can be used both to slide the patient across the bed and to turn the patient:

1. Slide the patient to one side of the bed.

2. Standing on the opposite side, draw the turning sheet over the patient's body, and gently roll the patient toward you, until the desired position is reached.

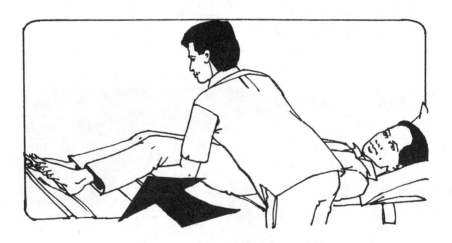

Figure 18

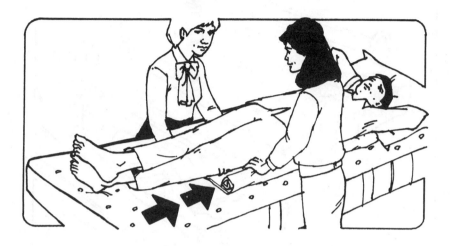

Figure 19

Changing Bed Linen

It is usual to change linen at the time that the patient bathes. However, perspiration or incontinence may require more frequent linen changes. If the patient is bed-ridden:

Procedure
1. Slide the patient to one side of the bed (Fig. 20).
2. Roll the soiled lower sheet toward the center of the bed and tuck well under the patient (Fig. 21).
3. Place the clean lower sheet, folded lengthwise, on the cleared section of the mattress, with the top section rolled toward the patient (Fig. 22).
4. With a turning sheet in place, roll the patient onto the freshly made part of the bed (Fig. 23).
5. Remove the soiled sheet and pull the fresh sheet tightly and tuck in (Fig. 24).
6. Replace the top sheet, leaving plenty of slack over the feet, so as to keep patient's feet comfortable.

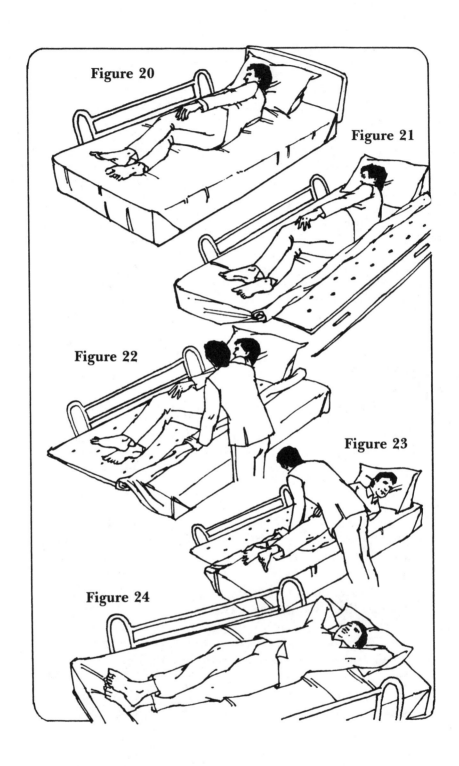

Figure 20

Figure 21

Figure 22

Figure 23

Figure 24

Patient Transfer to or from Bed

Procedure
1. Move the patient to the edge of the bed (see "Moving/Turning," p. 117) and into the side-lying position facing you.
2. Facing the head of the bed, place one foot in front of the other. Place one arm under the patient's shoulders and the other arm around him or her. Ask the patient to place the arm nearest you around your shoulders, and use the other arm to steady the patient against the mattress.
3. Brace your legs against the bed, and rock back, pulling the patient up and to you. The patient can assist by using the free arm and lowering his or her legs over the side of the bed (Fig. 25).

To move the patient to a bed-side chair or commode:
4. Place the chair close to the bed. If it is a wheel chair, lock the wheel.
5. Have the patient place his/her feet firmly on the floor, slightly apart.
6. Facing the patient, place his/her arms around your shoulders. Place your arms around the patient's back, clasping your hand (Fig. 26).
7. Brace yourself by placing your knees/thighs against those of the patient, and assist patient to balance as you rock patient forward to a standing position (Fig. 27).
8. Pivot the patient to the chair and lower the patient into the chair, bending at the knees to retain maximum support for both you and the patient, and sliding patient down into the chair (Figs. 28, 29).
9. Reverse this procedure to transfer the patient from a chair to the bed.

NOTE: This is a sensitive procedure, with potential for injury due to careless movements or sudden shifts of balance due to he patient's weakened condition. It is wise for team members to practice this procedure during team meetings to ensure that each team member is familiar with the procedure.

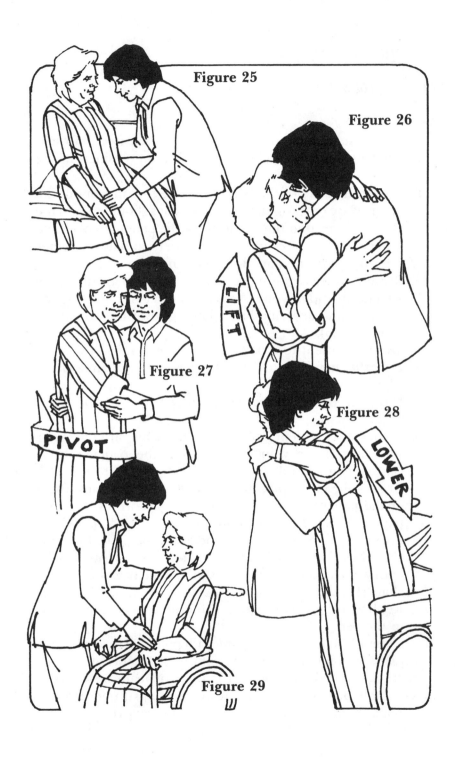

Figure 25

Figure 26

LIFT

Figure 27

PIVOT

Figure 28

LOWER

Figure 29

Infection Control

Patients will generally experience two concerns that may or may not be expressed directly, namely, protection of themselves from infections, and protection of those who are assisting them. They will expect helpers to exercise appropriate precautions when engaged in activities such as bathing, changing diapers, and other tasks. When handling body fluids, for example, you do not need to apologize for wearing gloves.

The AIDS virus is fragile, and has a short life outside its human host. It is not airborne. It is not transmitted by casual contact. Hugging, kissing, and touch are safe. Gloves are not indicated for normal household chores.

Danger of infection from team member to patient is a matter of much more urgency. It is advisable, therefore, to wash your hands thoroughly and frequently when engaged in patient care.

Investigation has demonstrated that even in hospital research laboratories or hospital rooms, danger of HIV infection to care providers is slight. Nevertheless, the team member should exercise common-sense precautions.

Procedure

1. It is best to remove jewelry (rings, watches) while caring for patients.
2. Protect yourself from patient's blood, urine, feces, vaginal discharges, and open wounds or sores by the use of latex gloves and hand-washing techniques.
3. Wear gloves when giving mouth care, bathing genitalia or rectal areas, or shaving the patient.
4. Wear gloves when handling items which have come in contact with blood, urine, feces, or sputum.
5. Remove soiled gloves before handling clean items.
6. Wear gloves at all times when changing diapers and cleaning the patient of any residual fecal material or blood.
7. Equipment (basins, urinals, bed pans, razors) should be rinsed with hot water after use. Items can be disinfected using a solution of one part bleach to ten parts water.
8. Clean surfaces that have been exposed to body fluids, using the 1:10 bleach solution; clean each surface twice.

9. Optional disposal of body waste: Prior to placing the patient on the bed-side commode or bed pan, you may set a plastic bag to collect feces for subsequent disposal. Soiled diapers similarly should be placed in a plastic bag for disposal. For added security, these items should be double-bagged.

Shaving

Team members may be called upon to shave men who are so weakened that they are unable to care for themselves. Patients who are able to communicate should be asked how they shave themselves and whether they want to do so with a team member's assistance. If the patient is unable to complete the task, the team member may do so. Since a longer beard is more difficult to shave, daily shaving is recommended. There appears to be no right or wrong way to perform this service for a patient. The following suggestions may make the task less difficult.

Procedure
1. Ensure that the room (or bed area) is well lit.
2. Electric razors may lessen the likelihood of cutting the patient, but many men prefer a blade shave. When shaving with a blade, use a fresh, clean blade.
3. Wash the patient's face with soap and warm water, rinse, dry, and apply warm water a second time.
4. Apply shaving cream thinly over the beard; if the cream is applied too thickly, it is difficult to see the skin as it is contoured over facial and jaw bones. Emaciated patients may have prominent facial bones, which will require special care as the skin surface is shaved.
5. Short, firm strokes with the razor seem to work well. Rinse the blade after each stroke.
6. After completing the shave, rinse the patient's face with clean warm water and apply after-shave lotion, if available.

THE JOURNEY CONTINUES . . .

If you have joined an AIDS Care Team, or are about to set out on this journey, we welcome you to the road and the journey. It is a long road, and we do not yet have the end in sight. You will find support along the way, from your congregation, other team members, your pastor, and, especially, from the people with AIDS and their families whom you will befriend, and who will become your guides. Expect to learn from them, to be inspired by them, and to be strengthened by their courage and fortitude.

BUT REMEMBER . . .

You are only human! There will be moments when you may wonder if you can keep going, or you feel like walking away from the responsibilities you accepted as a Care Team member. It is certainly appropriate to take a "sabbatical" and you may arrange to do so, in consultation with your team leader. However, you will often find that simply sharing your feelings with your pastor, team leader, or other team members is usually sufficient to help you deal with your ambivalence and grief, and at times, your anger and frustration.

The road will lead through dark valleys, sometimes desert plains that seem endless, but look up. The road lifts toward heights, and your soul will lift with the road.

EPILOGUE

The dedication of our volume *AIDS and the Church* (1987) closed with the prayer: "May this book soon be of historical interest only." The book recognized that AIDS is an unparalleled crisis, and the operative terms for each religious community were and still are *urgency, challenge, opportunity,* and *task*.[1] The crisis has arisen because of the stigma that attaches to HIV disease and its potential to destroy lives and communities: It is a situation that cries out for a redemptive response. As the people of God we dare not turn our backs.

Pastoral care-givers ministering to people living with HIV disease have begun to alert their peers in the pastoral care movement and in the religious community generally that we are confronted with a crisis of unprecedented proportions. The mortality rate for AIDS patients, the unremitting grief that accompanies care of this population, and the intensity of stigma associated with both the disease and people infected by the human immunodeficiency virus are contributing to the perception that AIDS is different from other diseases in new and troubling ways.[2] Response to people living with HIV disease is no longer a concern for a dedicated clergy and laypeople, but increasingly will be a mandate for every pastoral care-giver.

AIDS is not just one more disease entity in a long progression of terminal diseases to strike the human community. This disease differs from other diseases and places a new set of demands upon us. Consequently, *pastoral* care for people with AIDS can be assumed to thrust a new set of pastoral tasks upon the religious community.[3] This is particularly so in our response to the grief of people with AIDS: patients, families, partners, friends, and society. Elizabeth Goss proposes, for example, that as this predominantly young population of patients faces death, its members are evoking new perceptions about what it is like to die at the height of one's productive life, before life with its opportunities is fully realized.[4]

Maintaining openness to the depths of grief and joy occasioned by HIV disease is a work of unsurpassed intensity. At no time in the modern era have communities been called upon to marshall their resources to cope with an illness that is destroying thousands of people between birth and middle age, for which as yet there are few signs that relief is in sight. Our only indications are that the crisis has yet to reach its ultimate intensity. As the people of God, we are in this for the long haul.

We began this volume with a recognition that it is a partial, oncomplete picture—like stopping a movie and examining just one frame. Now the film sequence begins again, as each of us continues in ministry with people living with AIDS.

We close this manual on a note of mingled sadness and joy. Sadness, because despite all the efforts of physicians and medical researchers, we seem far from a solution to many of the enigmas of AIDS: It remains a disease of terrifying symptoms and proportions, and is still regarded as terminal. Yet despite the lack of encouragement that the end is in sight, and, even more, the fear that the crisis might reach as yet unimaginable proportions, the ministry to people living with AIDS in local communities is a cause for joy and celebration.

First, it is moving to observe and celebrate the steadfastness and courage of people with AIDS to whom the Care Teams in Houston minister. The measure of hope with which they face AIDS, and their decisions to meet life-threatening events head-on and claim victory over them, rather than admit defeat or live as "victims," is a inspiration and challenge to all of us.

Second, as the staff of the AIDS Interfaith Council participate in the recruitment, training, and daily ministries of the Care Teams, we are moved by the self-giving and commitment manifested by team leaders and by the members whose ministries they direct. We are moved even more by the warmth and beauty of the relationships that have been born between the people living with AIDS and the team members who serve them.

It is of the nature of the people of God to respond with warm and loving compassion to the needs of fellow human beings. In the urgency of the crisis that is exploding around us as the AIDS pandemic spreads, God's people are faced with challenges and tasks for which there are few precedents. But "challenges" and "tasks" are just other ways of talking about opportunities, and opportunities are calls to service and commitment. As servants of God, we live in a covenant with God, who assigns our work and to whom we are accountable for the proper discharge of our service.

And what is our service?

We are called to love the lord our God with all our hearts, and with all our minds, and with all our souls, and with all our strength . . .

and our neighbors as ourselves. (Deut. 6:5 and Lev. 19:18, paraphrase).

NOTES

1. Earl E. Shelp and Ronald H. Sunderland, *AIDS and the Church* (Philadelphia: The Westminster Press, 1987).
2. See Ronald H. Sunderland, "AIDS: Some Issues for Pastoral Care-givers," *The Journal of Pastoral Care*, 43 (Winter, 1989), pp. 293-95.
3. Ibid.
4. Elizabeth Goss, "Living and Dying with AIDS," *The Journal of Pastoral Care* 43 (Winter, 1989), pp. 297-308.

APPENDIX ONE

Adult AIDS Care Team Orientation

This program takes 7–8 hours, including lunch. Usually done in one day (Saturday). Teams typically have a brief meeting on another day to organize (select leaders, set geographical boundaries, establish pairs for visitation, set meeting dates, etc.).

I. Introduction
   A. AIDS: A challenge to God's people
   B. How local congregations are meeting this challenge
   C. Welcome to this dynamic and rewarding ministry

II. Paired exercises
   A. Previous experience with AIDS
   B. Why do you want to care for people with AIDS?
   C. Report to group

III. AIDS 101
   A. Epidemiology: U.S., state, and local projections
   B. HIV and modes of transmission
   C. AIDS: diagnostic criteria, clinical features
   D. Treatments and vaccines

IV. Psychosocial Features: HIV-seropositive person
   A. Unexpected disruption, uncertainty, threatened loss of plans, hopes
   B. Fear, stigma, alienation, secrecy
   C. Isolation and dependency
   D. Interpersonal and financial impact

V. Psychosocial Features: Family
   A. Awareness of risk factor of infected member

    B. Unexpected disruption, uncertainty, threatened loss of plans, hopes
    C. Fear, stigma, alienation, secrecy
    D. Isolation and altered roles
    E. Potential financial impact

  VI. Psychosocial Features: Lover
    A. Unexpected disruption, uncertainty, threatened loss of plans, hopes
    B. Fear, stigma, alienation, secrecy
    C. Isolation and preoccupation with care for lover
    D. Concern for self and relationships

  VII. Psychosocial Features: Intravenous Drug Users
    A. Confronting the client with substance abuse problems
    B. Behavioral manifestations of addiction
    C. Substance abuse as a multi-dimensional problem: physical, emotional, financial, legal
    D. Substance abuse as a "moral concern"
    E. Denial problems in substance users
    F. Co-dependency in AIDS

  VIII. Psychosocial Features: Hemophilia-related AIDS
    A. Infection traced to dependence on use of blood products and on the medical and scientific professions
    B. Distrust of the medical profession
    C. Teenage adjustment to hemophilia-related AIDS

  IX. Psychosocial Features: Blood Transfusion-related AIDS
    A. Heightened grief-related anger or depression
    B. Concern for privacy, confidentiality, withdrawal from customary support system
    C. Fear of loss of security and family and social relationships

X. AIDS Care Team Ministry
   A. Extension of ministry of God's people to the sick
   B. Respond to social, emotional, physical, and spiritual needs of people living with HIV disease
   C. Compassionate, non-judgmental, supportive
   D. Respect for people and unconditional love: spiritual and moral agenda to be set by client
   E. Empower people to retain control of life

XI. Lay Pastoral Ministry in the AIDS Care Team
   A. Ministry of listening and befriending activities as means to build relationships
   B. Message: "What happens to you matters to me."
   C. Mode: Be a story listener
   D. Grief results from changed perception of world due to sudden events that are experienced as losses
   E. Stories are means by which people invite others into their lives
      1. Stories cannot be forced
      2. Stories are told when people trust and sense one cares enough to listen
   F. Stories include facts and convey feelings
      1. Facts are vehicles for sharing feelings
      2. The listener's task is to listen and respond to feelings
      3. Listeners should not be tempted to counsel, which requires professional training
   G. There are two costs of caring:
      1. It takes *time* to listen
      2. The readiness to be *vulnerable*—to enter into another's pain
   H. Listening requires self-discipline:
      1. To avoid attempts to solve other people's problems
      2. To avoid assuming responsibility for other people or their circumstances
   I. Setting Limits
      1. A person in crisis may be tempted to dump

everything on a person who is trusted and perceived as non-exploitive and loving

2. Care-givers must learn to leave all this behind, continue their own lives, and do so without feeling guilty

3. Only by keeping adequate distance as a part of caring for themselves can care-givers go back repeatedly to face and share in the crises of others

J. Benefit to Clients

    1. Client learns to gain and exercise control

    2. Client is empowered to maintain autonomy, and avoid over-dependence

XII. Basic Physical Care

    A. Skills taught may be used only infrequently, and towards the end of life of the patient

    B. Asepsis and hygiene

    C. Temperature Control

    D. Movement and mobility

    E. Medications

    F. Death at home

XIII. Care Team Structure

    A. Service Coordinator and teams

    B. Team leaders and referral process

    C. Team members and client visitation

    D. Meetings, self and peer care, and staff support

    E. Accountability, reports

    F. Team meetings:

        1. Reports of team member activities

        2. Oversight (supervision) as the basis of continuing education

        3. In-service education, AIDS information up-dates

XIV. Conclusion

    A. Ministry as blessing

   B. Ministry as opportunity for self-growth and spiritual
      formation
   C. Ministry as a dynamic learning process
   D. Paired exercises:
      1. How has your thinking about AIDS changed?
      2. Report to group

Pediatric AIDS Family Care Team Orientation

This program takes 4 hours and should be given in addition to and following the orientation for care of adults.

I. Introduction
   A. Adaption of adult Care Team
   B. Similarities and differences

II. Paired Exercises: AIDS
   A. Why do you want to care for people with AIDS?
   B. Why do you want to care for children with AIDS?
   C. What do you think will differentiate adult care from child care?
   D. Report to group

III. Paired Exercises: Childhood illnesses
   A. Previous involvement with serious childhood illnesses or death, and its effect on you
   B. What do you anticipate you will feel from caring for pediatric AIDS families?
   C. Report to group

IV. Social Features
   A. People of Color
   B. Varied family structures
   C. Poverty
   D. Low level of education
   E. Possible correlation with chemical substance abuse
   F. Often transient families
   G. Access to phone and transportation
   H. Health status of parent(s): one or both may be HIV-seropositive, be diagnosed with AIDS, or face other health problems
   I. Information given to siblings: what they know or are to be told

V. Personal, Emotional, Psychological Features
  A. General perinatal transmission
    1. Poor communication skills
    2. Diverse value systems
    3. Suspicious of authority figures; coping skills may be manipulative
    4. Concern for privacy, confidentiality
    5. Guilt
    6. Physical and emotional fatigue
  B. Hemophilia-related AIDS
    1. Medically sophisticated
    2. Oriented to self-care
    3. High expectations of physicians, social services
    4. Higher level of education
    5. More access to health care, social services
    6. Concern for secrecy, confidentiality
    7. Feel victimized, angry
    8. Issues of sexuality and mortality among adolescents

VI. Special Features
  A. 1. Anticipated loss of child, or parent's own death
    2. Grief over being unable to watch child grow up
    3. Guilt at leaving child parentless
    4. Questions about how to inform *children* about parent's or child's illness
    5. Managing family conflict and disruptions related to AIDS
    6. Planning for care when parents no longer able to provide care
    7. Custody and estate planning
  B. Repeat pregnancy and decision to carry to term; possible reasons:
    1. Desire for child
    2. Religious belief
    3. Family pressure
    4. Fear of abandonment

        5. Withdrawal of financial support
        6. Physical violence
        7. Legacy
        8. Evidence of love for partner
   C. Personal Issues for Care Team Members
        1. Fear of contagion vs. impulse to hug and kiss
        2. Denial that HIV affects one's own social group (heterosexual, or women)
        3. Discomfort with sexuality or drug involvement
        4. Helplessness and despair in the client family because physical and social factors seem beyond control
        5. Anger and blame of the parent(s)
        6. Propensity to moralize
        7. Fear of personal adequacy

VII. Clinical Features of Pediatric AIDS patients
   A. Failure to thrive
   B. Developmental delay
   C. Organomegaly
   D. Hyperactivity
   E. Nutritional deficits
   F. Lymphadenopathy
   G. Chronic infections (other than AIDS-related opportunistic infections)
   H. Ear infections
   I. Diarrhea
   J. Pain (oral, cramps)

VIII. Nursing skills
   A. Washing
   B. Wound care (skin lesions)
   C. Oral care
   D. Play therapy (stimulation)
   E. Nutrition (normal diet, infant formula)
   F. Medications

IX. Guidelines for Care Team Members
- A. Remember that children with AIDS are children first, then children with illness
- B. Respect the parent-child bond, and parental roles and authority
- C. Make a clear contract with parents, e.g., time limits, functions
- D. Limits on specific family members who are to receive care
- E. Set limits to protect from over-identification
- F. Tolerate differences between yourself and the client family
- G. Maintain a strong level of self-esteem
- H. The goal of care is normalization and mainstreaming for child(ren) with AIDS
- I. Adopt and maintain realism about the future
- J. Develop and maintain openness and acceptance of expression of feelings
- K. Empower family to develop autonomy and control skills
- L. Be sensitive to needs and feelings of siblings
- M. Recognize and acknowledge support needs of extended family
- N. Plan care for survivors following death of family member with AIDS
- O. Use the Care Team processes to anticipate and provide for support needs of Care Team members before and following death of child(ren) or parent(s)

X. Paired exercise
- A. How has your thinking changed about pediatric AIDS care?
- B. Report to group

APPENDIX TWO

REPORT:_____ STATUS OF CLIENT:_____ Date:_____

Currently assigned to team:_____

Title:_____ First:_____ Last:_____ MI:_____

Sex:_____ Race:_____ Born:_____ (MM/DD/YY) SSN:_____

Address:_____

City:_____ State:_____ Zip:_____

Home phone: (____) _____-_____ Work Phone: (____) _____-_____

Intake on:_____ (MM/DD/YY) Assigned to team on:_____ (MM/DD/YY)

Keymap:_____ Emergency contact:_____

Comment:_____

Diagnosis code: • • • • • AIDS Transmission Category: • • • (see codes below)

HEALTH CARE RESOURCES
= = = = = = = = = =

Medicaid :   **MM** - Male to Male
VA   :   **IV** - IV drug use
County :   **MI** - Male to Male with IV drugs
Champus: **HM** - Hemophilia
COBRA :   **HS** - Heterosexual Sex
HMO   :   **TT** - Transfusion/Tissue
Self Pay :   **MR** - Mother infected/at Risk
Pvt. Ins. : COMMENT: **OU** - Other/Undetermined
Other   : EXPLAIN

Home Nursing:

Medically Indigent? :_____ As of:_____/_____/_____ (MM/DD/YY)

Medical contact:_____

Client referred by:_____(see codes at right)   **SE** - Self
     NU - Nurse
Referral Contact:_____   **PH** - Physician
     HN - Home Nursing Service
     SW - Social Worker
Referral Phone: (____) _____-_____   **OU** - Other/Undetermined

Other caretakers in home:_____ Minors in home:_____

Disposition:_____(Death, Refused by client, Needs met, Moved, Hold, Other)

Disposition Date:_____ (MM/DD/YY)

= = = = SUPPLY DATA ON CARE PROVIDED BETWEEN _____

AND _____ = = = =

HOURS OF CLIENT CARE _____.____

Team-Client Covenant

It is important that each team has a clear understanding with its clients concerning the activities team members are able to undertake. When this relationship is ambiguous and expectations on the part of each are unclear, frustration and anger often ensue. Nevertheless, it is difficult to propose a clear-cut covenant because the team may vary its agreement from client to client, and the team may amend its agreement with a particular client over a period of time as a client's needs and capacity for self-help change. The following suggestions may guide teams in adopting covenants with clients.

1. Teams may contract to offer specific services, for example:
   a. Social visits and outings
   b. Assisting client to shop for supplies; frequency may be indicated
   c. Transportation to physician's office, clinic, or other medical needs
   d. House cleaning
   e. Laundry
   f. Providing meals
   g. Sitting with client so a family member may go out

2. Teams may limit commitments or exclude specific services that members are unable or unwilling to undertake, for example:
   a. Providing financial support
   b. Purchasing medical/pharmaceutical supplies
   c. Limiting the frequency regarding 1 [g] above (e.g., once or twice per month)

d. Sitting with a client later than a specified time (e.g., 10.00 p.m.)

e. Sitting with client overnight

3. Where there is a primary care-provider (e.g., parent or lover), many problems due to misunderstandings, questions about who has authorized the team's ministry, or the extent of the team's ministry, may be avoided by ensuring that the care-provider either is included in the covenant-making or at least is informed of the agreement between the client and the Care Team. The team leader would insist that the team is present at the invitation of the client, and is responsible to the client as long as he or she is mentally competent.

4. In some instances, a team may covenant with a primary care-provider. For example, the care-provider may be physically or emotionally exhausted and be in need of respite from prolonged, intensive care of the person with AIDS, although the client has refused to accept direct care from the Care Team. In this case, the team may agree with the care-provider to sit in the home but not make direct contact with the client unless the client expresses need for assistance.

5. While we do not suggest we have exhausted all the possibilities, still less have all the answers, we will be pleased to respond to questions that interfaith councils or service coordinators may direct to us. We can be reached by phone at (713) 667-5627.

BIBLIOGRAPHY

Altman, Dennis, *AIDS in the Mind of America: The Social, Political, and Psychological Impact of a New Epidemic* (Garden City, N.J.: Anchor Press, 1886).

American Lutheran Church, The, "AIDS: A Serious and Special Opportunity for Ministry," *Mission Discoveries* 12 (July, 1987).

Amos, William E., Jr., *When AIDS Comes to Church* (Philadelphia: Westminster Press, 1988).

Confronting the AIDS Crisis, a Manual for Synagogue Leaders. Available from UAHC, 838 5th Avenue, New York, N.Y. 10021.

Edison, Ted, editor, *The AIDS Care Giver's Handbook* (New York: St. Martin's Press, 1988).

Fee, Elizabeth and Fox, Daniel M., editors, *AIDS: The Burdens of History* (Berkeley: University of California Press, 1988).

Flynn, Eileen P., *AIDS: A Catholic Call for Compassion* (Kansas City, Mo.: Sheed and Ward, 1985).

Fortunato, John E., *AIDS: The Spiritual Dilemma* (New York: Harper and Row, 1987).

Goss, Elizabeth, "Living and Dying with AIDS," *The Journal of Pastoral Care* 43 (Winter, 1989), 297-308.

Green, Ronald, "The Perspective of Jewish Tradition," *Religious Education* 83 (Spring, 1988), 221-32.

Kavar, Louis F., *Pastoral Ministry in the AIDS Era: Focus on Families and Friends of Persons with AIDS* (Wayzata, Minn.: Woodland Publishing Company, 1988).

Kirkpatrick, Bill, *AIDS: Sharing the Pain, A Guide for Care Givers* (New York: The Pilgrim Press, 1990).

Kirp, David L., *Learning by Heart: AIDS and School Children in America Communities* (New Brunswick: Rutgers University Press, 1989).

Kübler-Ross, Elisabeth. *AIDS: The Ultimate Challenge* (New York: Macmillan, 1987).

Melton, J. Gordon, *The Church Speaks on AIDS* (New York: Gale Research Inc., 1989).

Menz, R. L., "Aiding Those with AIDS: A Mission for the Church," *Journal of Psychology and Christianity* 6 (Fall, 1987), 5-18.

Moffat, B. C., editor, *AIDS: A Self-Care Manual* (Santa Monica: AIDS Project Los Angeles, IBS Press, 1987).

Monette, Paul, *Borrowed Time: An AIDS Memoir* (San Diego: Harcourt Brace Jovanovich, 1888).

Nelson, J. B., "Responding to, Learning From AIDS," *Christianity and Crisis* 46 (May 19, 1986), 176-81.

Peabody, Barbara, *A Mother's Journal of Her Son's Struggle with AIDS—A True Story of Love, Dedication and Courage* (San Diego: Oak Tress Publications, 1986).

Phillips, Jennifer, "The Future of AIDS: Parishes Can Help," *Christian Century* (June 1, 1988), pp. 548-51.

Richardson, Diane, *Women and AIDS* (New York: Methuen, 1989).

Sabatier, Renee, *Blaming Others: Prejudice, Race and Worldwide AIDS* (Washington, D.C.: The Panos Institute, 1988).

Shelp, Earl E., and Sunderland, Ronald H., editors, *A Biblical Basis for Ministry* (Philadelphia: Westminster Press, 1981).

Shelp, Earl E., and Sunderland, Ronald H., editors, *The Pastor as Prophet* (New York: The Pilgrim Press, 1985).

Shelp, Earl E., and Sunderland, Ronald H., editors, *The Pastor as Servant* (New York: The Pilgrim Press, 1986).

Shelp, Earl E., and Sunderland, Ronald H., editors, *The Pastor as Priest* (New York: The Pilgrim Press, 1987).

Shelp, Earl E., and Sunderland, Ronald H., editors, *The Pastor as Theologian* (New York: The Pilgrim Press, 1988).

Shelp, Earl E., and Sunderland, Ronald H., editors, *The Pastor as Teacher* (New York: The Pilgrim Press, 1989).

Shelp, Earl E., and Sunderland, Ronald H., editors, *The Pastor as Counselor* (New York: The Pilgrim Press, forthcoming).

Shelp, Earl E., "AIDS, High Risk Behaviors, and Moral Judgments," *The Journal of Pastoral Care* 43 (Winter, 1989), 325-35.

Smith, Walter J., *AIDS: Living and Dying with Hope, Issues and Pastoral Care* (New York: Paulist Press, 1988).

Sontag, Susan, *AIDS and Its Metaphors* (New York: Farrar, Strauss and Giroux, 1989).

Sunderland, Ronald H., "Caring for People Living and Dying with AIDS," *The Journal of Pastoral Care* 43 (Winter, 1989), 311-23.

Sunderland, Ronald H., "Working Through Your Grief: Picking Up the Pieces," VHS videotape, available from Service Corporation International, P.O. Box 12548, Houston, TX 77019.

Turner, Charles F., Miller, Heather G., and Moses, Lincoln E., editors, *AIDS: Sexual Behavior and Intravenous Drug Use* (Washington, D.C.: National Academy Press, 1989).

Wendler, K., "Ministry to Patients with Acquired Immunodeficiency Syndrome: A Spiritual Challenge," *Journal of Pastoral Care* 41 (March, 1987), 4-16.